Clinical Operation Techniques of Tooth Bleaching

（English－Chinese）

牙齿漂白临床实用手册

Editor in chief ◎ Meng Chao   Shen Jian   Kuang Xiaoming

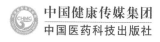

中国健康传媒集团

中国医药科技出版社

FOREWORD

With the continuous development of society, medical technologies and medical concepts are constantly updated, people have more demands on esthetic of dental restorations, tooth discoloration has become a problem that must be solved. More and more patients are requesting bleaching to improve the color of their teeth. Although there are many treatments available to improve tooth color in the era of all-porcelain restoration technology, the trauma caused by it is irreversible and inescapable. As patients and physicians seek noninvasive treatment techniques, there is a renewed emphasis and growth in tooth bleaching.

With the development of modern science and technology, the technology and concept of tooth bleaching are constantly updated. The application of different concentrations of bleaching agents, desensitization agents, electronic colorimeter and cold light bleaching instrument increases the success rate of tooth bleaching. The high success rate of tooth bleaching technology is helpful for clinicians to better treat discolored teeth.

This book systematically describes the clinical operation techniques of tooth bleaching, hoping to provide guidance and help for clinicians to carry out this technique more widely.

Meng Chao

May 2022

CONTENTS

7 Chapter 7 Home Bleaching Treatment Steps

8 Chapter 8 Complications

9 Chapter 9 Special Cases

10 Chapter 10 Postoperative Management

INTRODUCTION

With a history of nearly 145 years, tooth bleaching is a very popular and basic clinical practice. This technology should be taken seriously, neither "mythologized" nor "trivialized". From an indication point of view, the actual proportion of bleached teeth is quite large. Therefore, as a dental practitioner, we should understand and standardize the mastery of this technique.

Our team has accumulated a lot of clinical experience and knowledge, and we have hired 12 doctors and scholars with rich experience in the field as consultants to systematically explain the process and precautions of tooth bleaching. The cases in the book are the accumulation of front-line clinical cases over many years. It is hoped that this book will provide help for peers on how to develop and view this technology in a correct and standardized way.

"Clinical Operation Techniques of Tooth Bleaching" is a graphic interpretation of the standardized operation of tooth bleaching. We believe that it can play a positive role in helping clinicians to treat tooth discoloration.

Chapter 1
Tooth Discoloration

Normal teeth are shiny yellowish white. Changes in tooth color due to changes in the body or inside the teeth are called tooth discoloration, also known as endogenous tooth coloration. Tooth coloring caused by the deposition of pigments carried or produced by bacteria entering the oral cavity on the tooth surface is called exogenous tooth coloration.

Tooth discoloration includes but not limited to discoloration of individual teeth caused by local factors and discoloration of multiple teeth or whole teeth caused by systemic factors, such as tetracycline pigmentation teeth, dental fluorosis, etc.

Exogenous tooth coloration refers to external tooth coloration related to lifestyle, such as food, drink or tobacco. Some drugs carry ingredients that can also cause coloration, such as Tin(II)Fluoride, chlorhexidine, etc. With the change of age, the sensitivity of teeth to exogenous coloration increases continuously. Exogenous coloration often coexists with salivary protein film, dental plaque or dental calculus on the tooth surface.

1 The cause of discoloration

Tooth discoloration is a complex physical and chemical process. The combination of colored substances and tooth tissues in physiological or pathological states leads to tooth discoloration. Causes are as follows:

(1) Pulp bleeding

Dental pulp blood vessel rupture caused by dental trauma or the use of arsenic deactivated pulp, or because of excessive bleeding during mechanical pulp extraction, the decomposition of blood products, infiltration into the dentin tubules, causing the surrounding dentin discoloration. The degree of discoloration increases with time. In the early stage of pulp hemorrhage due to trauma, the crown appears pink. The blood penetrates into the pulp wall and reaches the dentin layer. Later, the crown may appear light gray, light brown or grayish brown.

(2) Pulp necrosis

The dead pulp of the tooth produces hydrogen sulfide, which reacts with hemoglobin to form black iron sulfide. Melanin can also come from melanin-producing pathogens. Black material slowly seeps into the dentin tubules and the teeth appear grayish black or black.

(3) Excessive calcification of dentin

After trauma, irregular dentin formed along the wall of the root canal in the medullary cavity, resulting in decreased transparency of the crown and yellow or yellowish brown discoloration.

(4) Dietary sources

Food, beverages, areca nuts and tobacco have a cumulative discoloration effect. Especially enamel and dentin crack, wear of the elderly more obvious.

(5) Dehydration of dentin

The nonvital teeth lose their nutritional support from the pulp, and dehydration of dentin causes the surface of the teeth to lose its translucent luster and take on a dull gray color.

(6) Medical factors

- Residual pulp: The discoloration is caused by the gradual decomposition of the pulp left during root canal treatment.
- Drugs or filling materials used in the cavity and root canal, such as iodide and chlortetracycline, can turn the teeth into light yellow, light brown or light gray; silver amalgam and copper amalgam can make the teeth around the filling black; phenolic resin can make teeth reddish brown, etc.

2 Classification of discoloration

Healthy natural teeth are not uniform in color, but show gradual changes in color at the neck, body, and incisors due to differences in enamel and dentin thickness, light reflection, and transparency.

Because different tooth discoloration has different sensitivity to bleaching treatment, it is necessary to carefully evaluate the types and causes of tooth discoloration in order to develop a sound bleaching treatment plan and achieve good bleaching results.

The types of tooth discoloration can be divided into exogenous and endogenous discoloration.

(1) Exogenous discoloration is a staining substance that affects the enamel surface. The categories are as follows:

- Living habits

People who drink tea, coffee, smoke tobacco products or chew areca for a long time will have brown or dark-brown staining on the surface of their teeth, especially on the tongue, which cannot be removed by brushing. The grooves and rough surfaces of teeth are also easy to stain.

- Poor oral hygiene

The external pigments were first deposited in the mucous membrane and plaque of the tooth surface. In people with poor oral hygiene, plaque remains, such as near the gingival margin, where the adjacent surface is often stained. As the plaque demineralize the surface of the tooth, the pigment can also seep into the tooth tissue.

- Medicine

Long-term use of chlorhexidine, potassium permanganate solution gargle or use pharmaceutical toothpaste, such as chlorhexidine toothpaste, can have light brown or dark brown coloring on the surface of teeth; When the teeth are treated locally with ammonia silver nitrate, the corresponding parts will turn black.

- Occupational exposure

Occupational contact due to the need to contact some minerals, such as iron, sulfur, teeth can be brown; contact with copper, nickel, chromium, etc., teeth surface may appear green deposits.

- Other factors

The viscosity, pH of saliva and the growth of pigmentation bacteria carried or produced in oral cavity are related to exotic pigment deposition. The change of age also increases the sensitivity of teeth to exogenous coloration.

(2) Endogenous discoloration is the discoloration of tooth structure, which is classified as follows:

- The etiology comes before the teeth burst out, such as blood disorders, the enamel and dentin not well developed, etc.
- The etiology comes from the period of tooth development, such as taking tetracycline, excessive intake of fluoride, etc.
- The etiology comes after the teeth have erupted, such as pulp necrosis, tooth trauma, dental caries, restorative materials and some dental procedures caused by various factors, as well as age-related changes of some teeth (thinning of enamel, secondary increase of dentin, etc.)

| Chapter 2
| Tooth Bleaching
| Techniques

Bleaching is a method of lightening teeth by using chemicals to oxidize the organic pigments in the teeth. Compared with other aesthetic techniques to improve tooth color, bleaching treatment has the advantages of less trauma to the affected tooth, maximum retention of hard tissue integrity, and simple clinical operation. The disadvantages are that the treatment time is a little longer, the long-term duration of bleaching effect is not easy to predict, and the prognosis of some cases may not reach the expected effect of patients, which should be explained to patients before treatment.

1 Chemical reaction

Bleach is generally an oxidant. REDOX reaction occurred between bleach and discolored tooth tissue. Bleaching agents placed behind teeth release reactive oxygen species; through chemical reaction, the total amount of discoloration material is reduced and transformed into a colorless substance. Peroxide diffused into the dentin structure and reached the dentin around the tube, which was accompanied by oxidation reaction.

Enamel can be seen as a translucent membrane that allows bleach to penetrate into the teeth. The surface area of the enamel is important. Bleach is activated by complex oxidation reactions that release oxygen and other free radicals. Oxygen and other free radicals penetrate into the dentin through the gaps between the columns, thereby bleaching the teeth.

Bleach penetrates from the enamel to the dentin and pulp within 5-10 minutes of starting action. At the same time, bleach is easy to penetrate from the weakest places of teeth, such as cracks, cleavage planes, demineralized areas chalk spots and other poorly mineralized areas.

Bleaching is a very complex process that is affected by many factors, including: ① the pH of the bleaching agent; ② how and when to use bleach; ③ the change of illumination; ④ time of illumination; ⑤ selective absorption of light wavelength; ⑥ tooth structure.

2 Treatment objects

Depending on who is treated, tooth bleaching can be divided into vital teeth and nonvital teeth bleaching, both of which include clinic bleaching and household bleaching. As the name suggests, clinic bleaching is done by a physician in a clinic, while household bleaching is done at home with a low concentration of bleach after the patient leaves the clinic.

Whether it is clinic bleaching or household bleaching, it is necessary to correctly determine the cause of tooth discoloration before surgery, understand the patient's expectations, and fully communicate with the patient on the course of treatment, cost, expected effect and possible complications, so as to select and develop the best treatment plan and obtain close cooperation from the patient. During bleaching treatment, it is very important to record the color of teeth. The baseline value of the patient's color of teeth before bleaching was determined using a colorimeter or electronic colorimeter and recorded in the patient's presence. After bleaching treatment, the same colorimetric method was used again to determine the tooth color and record it. Additional records can also be obtained by taking close-up photos of the patient's teeth and smiling photos. All photos should be taken under the same environment, body position and magnification conditions, and the effect of bleaching can be evaluated by comparing the color of the teeth before and after bleaching.

3 Influencing factors

(1) Tooth surface cleaning

Thoroughly clean the tooth surface before bleaching to ensure that the bleach agent is in full contact with the tooth surface. Bleaching treatment is generally recommended to begin 2 weeks after dental scaling to reduce sensitivity and gum problems.

(2) Peroxide concentration

With the increase of peroxide concentration, oxidation enhanced, bleaching speed will accelerate. When using high concentrations of hydrogen peroxide, care should be taken to protect the gums from chemical burns.

(3) Temperature

The higher the temperature, the faster oxygen is released and the faster the color of your teeth changes. When temperatures rise to uncomfortable levels, tooth sensitivity and even irreversible pulpitis disease can occur.

(4) pH

Hydrogen peroxide helps maintain its potency during transportation and storage at acidic pH, while it works best during bleaching at pH 9.5 to 10.8.

(5) Time

The effect of bleaching is directly related to the time the bleaching agent is in contact with the tooth surface. Within a certain range, the longer the exposure time, the better the bleaching effect, but at the same time, the possibility of postoperative sensitization increases

(6) Storage environment

Keeping hydrogen peroxide in a closed environment maintains its bleaching efficiency.

Chapter 3
Materials and Equipment for Tooth Bleaching

1 Bleaching agents

Bleach is generally an oxidant. Common bleach agents include hydrogen peroxide, sodium perborate, and urea peroxide in various concentrations.

(1) Hydrogen peroxide

Hydrogen peroxide is the most effective bleaching agent and can be used in a variety of concentrations (3%-40%). Hydrogen peroxide is mainly used for bleaching outside the crown, but can also be used for bleaching inside the crown. However, it should be noted that high concentration of hydrogen peroxide is corrosive to soft tissue and will cause severe burning sensation after contact, so attention should be paid to protection during clinical use. High concentration of hydrogen peroxide is easy to decompose when heated and should be stored in cold storage away from light.

(2) Urea peroxide

Urea peroxide is relatively stable and can be decomposed to produce urea, ammonia, carbon dioxide and hydrogen peroxide. When decomposed, 10% urea peroxide can produce nearly 3.5% hydrogen peroxide. The common concentration is 5%-20%, which is irritating to the pulp and surrounding tissues, and is mainly used for bleaching outside the crown.

(3) Sodium perborate

Sodium perborate is an oxidant and can be made in a variety of dosage forms. Fresh sodium perborate contains 95% perborate and releases 9.9% oxygen. Dried sodium perborate is more stable and breaks down into sodium metaborate, water and eco-oxygen when exposed to acid, heat or water.

2 Common instruments

(1) Examination instruments

Examination instruments include oral scope, forceps, common probe, periodontal probe, weak straw, three-use gun barrel, patient protective glasses, drapes and mouthwash cup. (3-1 to 3-4)

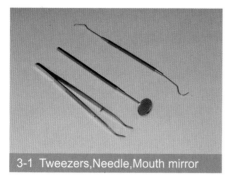
3-1 Tweezers,Needle,Mouth mirror

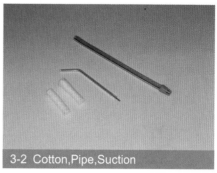
3-2 Cotton,Pipe,Suction

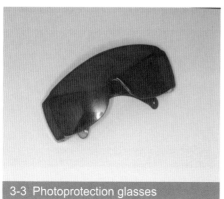
3-3 Photoprotection glasses

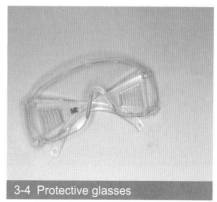
3-4 Protective glasses

(2) Preoperative instruments

Impression tray/oral scan protective cover, ultrasonic cleaner (including master machine and working tip), sandblasting machine, low-speed mobile phone (including rubber cup and polishing paste/pumice powder), colorimetric system (colorimetric plate/electronic colorimeter). (3-5 to 3-10)

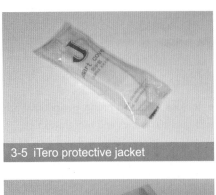

3-5 iTero protective jacket

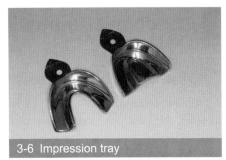

3-6 Impression tray

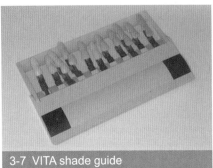

3-7 VITA shade guide

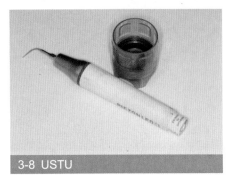

3-8 USTU

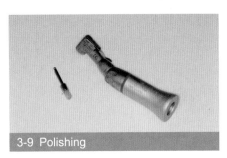

3-9 Polishing

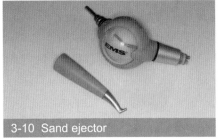

3-10 Sand ejector

(3) Surgical instruments

Mouth opener (including tongue block), lip balm, rubber dam, dental floss, wet cotton roll, gingival protector, light curing lamp, tooth bleach. (3-11 to 3-16)

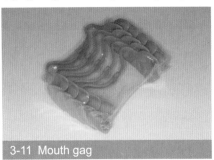

3-11 Mouth gag

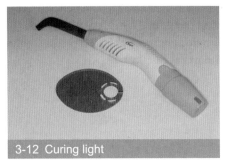

3-12 Curing light

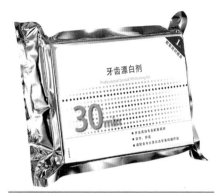

3-13 Teeth bleaching (Solo)

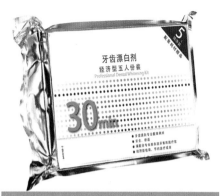

3-14 Teeth bleaching (5 people)

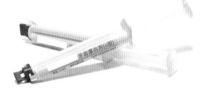

3-15 Decolorant

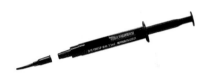

3-16 Gum protcetant

3 Common equipment

- Tooth bleaching machine.
- Electronic colorimeter.
- Oral scanner.
- Light curing lamp.
- Ultrasonic tooth cleaner.
- Sandblasting machine.

| Chapter 4
| Case Selection

1 Indications

There are a wide range of indications for tooth bleaching, including living teeth, nonvital teeth and special cases.

(1) Indications for bleaching of living pulp teeth

- Exogenous discoloration, the most important clinical case, mainly comes from the diet structure, such as tea, coffee, areca nut, tobacco products and dyeing condiments; drug staining such as long-term use of chlorhexidine or potassium permanganate mouthwash and toothpaste caused by staining.
- Excessive calcification of dentin.
- Aging results in increasing sensitivity of teeth to exogenous coloration.
- Poor oral hygiene.
- Occupational contact, dental staining due to contact with certain minerals at work.

(2) Indications for bleaching of nonvital teeth

- Pulp hemorrhage.
- Dentin dehydration.

(3) Special cases

- Hereditary amelogenesis imperfecta. (Chalky spots, white lines and other white lesions.)
  In some patients, enamel may be chalky, even cheesy, or hard. Bleaching is usually the first treatment for this type of tooth, and the chalky patches are removed after surgery, so there is no need for other treatment because bleaching is non-invasive. However, if the results are not satisfactory, the shape and color should be restored using a combination of micro-grinding techniques or dental prosthetics.
- Enamel development defects due to nutritional deficiency, febrile disease, and hypocalcemia.

Enamel development defects due to nutritional deficiency, febrile disease, and hypocalcemia: The concave surface of tooth enamel, where the concave is easy to stain. Usually for this kind of tooth bleaching treatment first, after the stain fades, do not need to receive other treatment;

- Dental fluorosis

Light or dark colored affected teeth without obvious defects can be bleached. However, the severely damaged teeth should be repaired by composite resin, porcelain, glass ceramic veneer or full crown.

- Tetracycline teeth

Tetracycline teeth are a special kind of discolored teeth. The staining area of tetracycline teeth is dentin, and bleach is not easy to reach the staining area through the enamel, so it is difficult to treat. For pale yellow discoloration cases and cases where the discoloration area is limited to the end of the incision, the effect is good, the prognosis of heavy gray black is poor, but most of them will improve, 80% of the cases can maintain the effect for more than 1 year. The obvious and effective decolorization method for tetracycline teeth is the coronal bleaching method, that is, the pulp is removed, the root is filled, the use of nonvital tooth bleaching technology, so that the drug directly acts on the discolored dentin. Although this method is obvious, but the side effects are also obvious, clinical caution. For moderately stained or severely enamel defect teeth can be repaired with porcelain, glass ceramic veneer or full crown, or can be first discolored and then covered restoration (but with the progress of color masking agent, this step may be eliminated in the future).

2 Contraindications

Absolute contraindications to bleaching are rare. Most contraindications are relative, usually related to anatomical conditions, oral health, and patient expectations.

(1) The anatomical structures involved in bleaching

- Deciduous/mixed dentition.
- Tooth cleft or pulp cavity is too large.
- Enamel hypoplasia.
- Local discoloration of teeth can be improved by filling prostheses.
- Limited surgical field of vision and surgical instruments due to local anatomical conditions: for example, limited opening can not effectively expose enough oral field of vision for operation; in addition, due to the limitations of visual field and device access, such as mouth opener and tongue block instability, often make a routine bleaching surgery difficult to perform.

(2) Oral health

- Patients with dentin allergy.

- Periodontal disease.
- The teeth have a large area of fillings and restorations.
- Pregnant women, lactating women and people allergic to chemical substances.

(3) Patient expectations

When patients lack correct understanding of tooth bleaching, including excessive requirements for color, strict guarantee for long-term results, and desire to compare bleaching with prostheses, it is necessary to carefully evaluate and grasp the risks of surgery. Patients with psychological disorders at the same time, if necessary, need to ask specialist consultation, give appropriate treatment, until the disease is stable and then choose the operation.

| Chapter 5
| Treatment Plan

The development of a treatment plan is an essential step in bleaching treatment, as bleaching treatment is often the beginning of a series of aesthetic treatments. Dental practitioners need to develop a detailed treatment plan for their patients. A treatment plan should be carefully developed to fully explain to the patient the principles of bleaching treatment, the necessary preliminary treatment to be completed before bleaching treatment and the considerations involved after bleaching treatment. Improving and maintaining oral health is a primary consideration.

Before evaluating the patient, the physician should understand the patient's oral health needs and requirements. Ask a new patient, "What problem would you most like to solve?" "What do you expect from your teeth?" Patients may have their own special thoughts and specific concerns, and wish to discuss and communicate with the physician. While some patients have Not considered it carefully before, others have their own dental "plan" containing areas they wish to improve and have a clear aesthetic need for improvement.

This section enumerates all aspects required for the development of a comprehensive treatment plan for tooth bleaching, describes how to carry out the bleaching plan, demonstrates methods of gathering information, and emphasizes the importance of systemic and dental history. Patient communication, smile analysis, patient expectations, informed consent were discussed. This section provides a practical questionnaire and form template that can be used in the information gathering phase.

1 Doctor-patient communication

Good and clear communication should be established with the patient before any dental treatment is performed. The physician must identify the needs of the patient in order to accurately understand the patient's concerns about tooth discoloration and the corresponding aesthetic needs. Beauty is an abstract subjective concept, but it is also an essential part of human nature. Culture, age, gender, occupation and time will affect patients' understanding of beauty. Considering this subjectivity, good communication between doctors and patients should be established at the beginning of treatment to work together towards the same goal.

Good communication can improve treatment acceptance. To achieve informed consent, patients need to understand the benefits, risks, advantages and disadvantages of treatment; Problems associated with refusing treatment; The importance of each treatment. The risks and benefits of treatment should be communicated to the patient before treatment begins. Good communication is especially important when patients' expectations exceed reality.

Patients' expectations for their own smiles can be assessed using questionnaires that include their self-perception of their own teeth and smile. The questions should be open-ended, allowing patients to express any concerns they may have. Questions can be asked about tooth shape, location, color and proportion. The information collected will be able to establish a baseline from which physicians can interact and communicate with patients to assess their aesthetic problems.

It is important to emphasize that patients should be asked about their expectations and perceptions of eventual treatment outcomes. A thorough dental and oral health assessment must be initiated before starting bleaching treatment. It is useful to use checklists to help gather information so that you have all the necessary information.

2 Scheme design and informed consent

(1) A list of new patients

The following information should be collected during each new patient's consultation:
- Informed consent to be examined.
- History of the whole body.
- Past dental treatment.
- External oral examination.
- Oral examination: soft tissue examination; Dentition examination; Periodontal examination; Occlusal examination; Temporomandibular joint function; Dental pulp vitality.
- Digital X-ray panoramic film.
- Other information: Research model/Oral scan electronic model; in-mouth camera photos.

(2) History of the whole body

The patient's overall condition should be carefully assessed. A history of chronic illness or long-term use of antibiotics (tetracycline, etc.) may cause tooth discoloration. Preterm infants may develop enamel dysplasia or chalk patches and white lesions on teeth. Patients should fill out a special bleaching questionnaire. The patient's diet should be assessed: smoking habits, drinking habits, chewing of betel nut, etc. Patients should change their diet during bleaching, such as quitting tobacco or cutting back on smoking.

Attention should be paid to whether the patient is allergic to plastics, peroxide, or other components contained in bleaching systems. Current medications, especially medications that may cause dry mouth, such as antihistamines, should be noted on the systemic history page. Patients taking hormones may occasionally develop excessive gingival edema. In view of the current lack of information on the effects of bleaching on the developing embryo, patients during pregnancy or breastfeeding should not receive bleaching treatment.

(3) Dental treatment history

Causes of tooth discoloration should be analyzed. Different causes (e.g., caries, internal absorption, external absorption, trauma, drugs, etc.) require different treatments.

Exogenous discoloration can usually be removed by sound dental professional cleaning (ultrasonic cleaning, sandblasting, low speed polishing).

(4) Smile analysis and aesthetics

What is a beautiful smile? One definition is that the size, position and color of the teeth are in harmony with each other, and the teeth are symmetrical and proportional to each other and in harmony with the surrounding tissue. Teeth are only part of the smile aesthetic, and should be viewed within the framework of the soft tissue of the gums, the buccal corridor area within the dental arch, and the lips and face.

Tooth bleaching may not meet all of a patient's needs. Smile analysis should be performed before bleaching treatment and should be included in the treatment planning stage. Smile analysis tables can be used to determine smile requirements and patient needs. Many factors need to be considered in smile analysis: tooth shape and length, lip line, smile line and occlusal relationship. Each of these factors is an important feature, all of them are woven together to achieve aesthetic harmony.

(5) Check in the sprue

Dental and periodontal conditions should be examined before bleaching treatment. Poor restorations should be recorded and discussed with the patient prior to treatment. The main areas to be assessed are:

- Enamel thickness.
- Gum height or amount of gum retreat.
- Tooth sensitivity: dentine sensitivity and cleft.
- Tooth permeability.
- Chalky or white lesions: will not disappear after treatment and may worsen in a short time.
- Banded discoloration: caused by tetracycline teeth or dehydration, it will still be banded after treatment and needs to be informed before surgery.
- Gingivitis: Gingivitis or periodontitis requires treatment first.
- Dehydration line: aging will lead to thinning of enamel, and the third stage of dentin deposition will lead to thickening of dentin and yellowing of teeth with aging. This process will produce dehydration line due to uneven, but also can Not evenly whiten, will show two colors along the dehydration line.
- Dark cracks and lesions: usually caused by smoking, betel nut and night grinding.

(6) Special inspections

- Pulp vitality test: hot and cold temperature test or electrical vitality test can be used.

- Imaging: As a general rule, apical films should be taken before all bleaching treatments. For pathological problems, dental caries, apical inflammation, etc., the best panoramic film screening; CBCT screening should be assisted in places with special diseases. Note that bleaching may induce acute episodes of periapical lesions, and discoloration of a single tooth may cause pulp death. These should be identified and screened before surgery.
- Intra oral digital image: it can record the preoperative status, which is very helpful for the analysis of dental caries, cracks, defects, restorations and tooth status.
- Diagnostic model: Due to the possibility of home bleaching treatment, personalized braces made from dentition models are required. The conventional methods are plaster after impression and 3D printing of oral scan data.

(7) There are old restorations in the aesthetic area

The patient must be informed in advance that although the old prostheses match the color of the teeth, the teeth are lighter after bleaching treatment and the old prostheses may need to be replaced for a better color match. The composite resin filling body does not change color due to bleaching. Sometimes bleaching treatments remove the discoloration at the edges of old restorations, thus making old restorations appear lighter. Bleaching treatment reduces enamel sensitivity to bonding treatment.

(8) The patient's expectations

Prior to any bleaching treatment, the patient's expectations must be assessed. Patients seeking "pure white teeth", "Hollywood whites" and "celebrity teeth" are rarely satisfied with bleaching treatments. A colorimeter can be used to explain the color changes to the patient before treatment. Patients should be aware that some teeth may not be bleached and some teeth may Not be evenly whitened. The darker the tooth, the longer it takes to bleach. Elderly patients near the root surface of bleaching effect is poor, the bleaching time is long. Treatment time and appointment arrangements are different for patients of different ages. Patients should be informed of this before bleaching treatment and should be informed of the risks of being near the root and neck of the tooth.

(9) Photo shoot of bleaching treatment

Standard photographic procedures must be followed to develop a treatment plan. The quality of the photos should be high, and SLR cameras should be used if conditions are available to achieve standardization. Preoperative and postoperative comparison photos should be taken. Digital photos can be cropped and easily standardized, facilitating the establishment of preoperative and postoperative comparison photo case library.

Patients often forget the color and discoloration of teeth before treatment, and photos can be a good reminder for patients to Notice changes in tooth color and avoid unnecessary disputes. A colorimetric plate can be used as a reference for preoperative photographs. Patients will recognize changes in their teeth when they see changes in the colorimetric number.

Bleaching treatment should be photographed.

Before and after treatment:
- Front view of the patient.
- Smile.
- Pull view.
- Place the color plate on the left maxillary cusp and take a smile picture.
- Black background pull view of anterior teeth.

(10) Treatment plan discussion and informed consent

Before starting any dental treatment, the treatment plan should be discussed with the patient. Patients can browse the whole situation of their mouth from the screen of the computer or mobile phone, and show patients the oral photos, electronic oral scan data, imaging examination data and plaster model, etc. The treatment plan, sequence of treatments and possible follow-up treatments need to be explained in detail to the patient. Communication is a two-way street, and the patient has the opportunity to ask further questions and clarify what is involved in the treatment plan, especially when it comes to home bleaching. The benefits and risks of treatment, as well as the advantages and disadvantages of treatment options, should be discussed with the patient, and options for bleaching or alternative therapies should be explained.

An informed consent form must be obtained, signed personally by the patient, in duplicate, one for the patient and one for retention in the patient's medical record. Informed consent should include all possible side effects.

(11) Color evaluation and color comparison

There are many methods for colorimetry before bleaching treatment, the more commonly used are traditional colorimetry and electronic colorimetry. Traditional color palette is more widely used, but more subjective; Electronic colorimeters are more accurate and controllable, but require additional delivery equipment.

We discuss the influence factors of traditional colorimetry: natural light during colorimetry; the hue of the teeth; The brightness of the teeth; The color of the teeth.

The study of tooth color and colorimetry is a broader topic, which will not be discussed in this paper. It is worth mentioning that clinical operations must be performed with and only one colorimetric system to achieve accuracy, proficiency and reproducibility. (5-1 to 5-17)

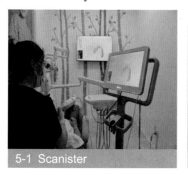

5-1 Scanister

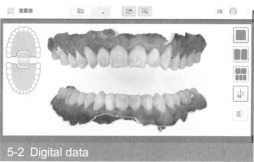

5-2 Digital data

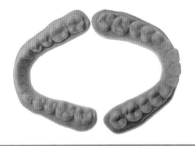

5-3 3D dental model 1

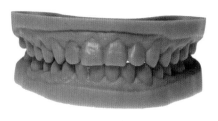

5-4 3Ddental model 2

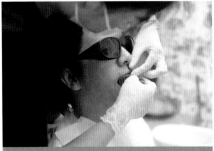

5-5 Try impression tray

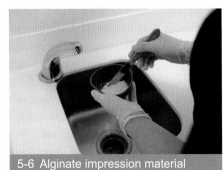

5-6 Alginate impression material

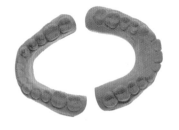

5-7 Copy teeth model

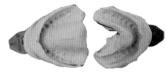

5-8 Alginate impression material model

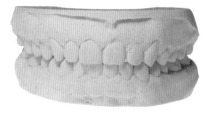

5-9 Plaster model 1

5-10 Plaster model 2

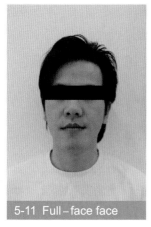
5-11 Full-face face

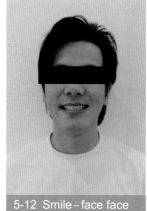
5-12 Smile-face face

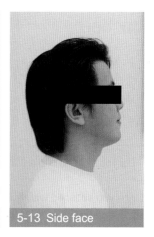
5-13 Side face

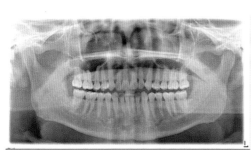
5-14 Orthopantomography X-ray

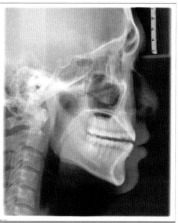
5-15 Lateral cephalometric X-ray

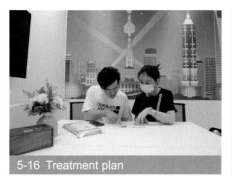
5-16 Treatment plan

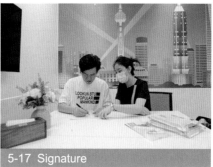
5-17 Signature

Attached:

XXXX Dental Outpatient Department
Smile evaluation scale

1. Do you like the current appearance (size and shape) of your teeth?	Yes ☐	No ☐
2. Are you satisfied with the current color of your teeth?	Yes ☐	No ☐
3. Do you want to whiten your teeth?	Yes ☐	No ☐
4. Are you satisfied with the uniformity of your teeth?	Yes ☐	No ☐
5. Do you have any missing teeth that you hope to be able to repair?	Yes ☐	No ☐
6. Do you have prostheses (silver amalgam fillings/metal crowns) that you wish to replace?	Yes ☐	No ☐

7. If you could change anything about your smile, what specific changes would you make?
Specific: _____

_____

_____

Preoperative Questionnaire for New Patients

Time of first diagnosis: _____

Name: _____

Date of birth: _____ Gender: ☐ Male ☐ female

Contact information: _____

Chief complaint:	
Which dental problems would you like to solve:	
Which treatments do you wish to receive:	
Your hopes and requirements for physicians:	

Anxiety and aversion associated with treatment:		
Previous dental treatment:	Last dental visit:	
	Regular follow-up:	
	Specific treatment:	
Pain or Not (specific nature):		
Sensitivity or Not (specific triggers):	☐ Hot ☐ sweet	☐ cold ☐ pressure other:
Gum problems:	☐ Bleeding ☐ redness	☐ stone ☐ atrophy other:
Previous oral hygiene maintenance and treatment:		
Smile line and lip line:		
What do you like most about your smile?		
What do you dislike most about your smile?		
What would you like to improve?		
Are you satisfied with the color of your teeth?		
Do you wish your teeth to be adducted or straightened?		
Do you have any hope of closing the tooth space?		
Are you satisfied with the uniformity of your teeth?		
Are you satisfied with the shape of your teeth?		
Do you have any hope of repairing the missing tooth?		

Do you have prostheses (silver amalgam fillings/metal crowns) that you wish to replace?	

Teeth:

Previous orthodontic treatment history:			
Food embedded plug:			
Wisdom teeth:			
Temporal-mandibular joint	☐ Snapping ☐ Bruxism ☐ Trismus ☐ Surgery		
Other Supplementary matters:			

Examination, diagnosis

Patient details:

Name:	Gender: ☐ Male ☐ female	Date of birth:
Mobile phone No.:	Email:	WeChat:
Expectations and requirements for tooth bleaching:		
General medical history (medication history) :		

Diagnosis of tooth discoloration:

Color type:	Mild	Moderate	Severe
The current color:		Desired color:	
☐ Chalk spots		☐ Fluorine spot tooth	
☐ Brown spots		☐ Tetracycline teeth	
☐ Dehydration lines		☐ Dark crack	
Others:			
Whether teeth are sensitive: ☐ Yes ☐ No		Do you have a history of dental sensitivities: ☐ Yes ☐ No	
Imaging and dental photographs:			

The date the image was taken:		Date of image reading:	
☐ Periapical film	☐ Panoramic X-ray	☐ Lateral projection	☐ CBCT
☐ Pictures inside the mouth Date of shooting:		☐ Pictures outside the mouth Date of shooting:	

Pulp vitality test:

Check in the sprue:

Gingival retreat:
In need of treatment:
Old restorations:

Periodontal disease: ☐ Yes ☐ No

The patient requires further repair and treatment as follows:

Physician's Signature:	Date:

Tooth bleaching Prescription

Bleaching treatment type:	Fundamental	Intermediate	Advanced
Date of general history review:		Date of medication history review:	
Current internal conditions:		Preoperative information and examination:	
Anterior tooth filling:		Gum condition:	Gingival recession:
Full crown:		Chalk spots:	Dark crack:
Full crown of implant:		Brown spots:	Tooth sensitivity:
Veneering:		The old filler:	Dehydration lines:
Others:		Restoration:	Tetracycline teeth:
		Dental fluorosis:	Others:
Clinic bleaching:		Household bleach:	

Tooth bleaching treatment products:

Product name	
Product concentration	
Desensitizer	
Disclaimer	
Date	

The patient was informed and consented to treatment:

Patient's signature:	Date:

treatment record:

Number of visits:	Time for follow-up visits:
Treatment plan:	
Date of last visit:	Date of final photo taken:

The final color:

Informed Consent Form/Health Record Form For Dental Bleaching Patients

DATE: _____ / _____ / _____   Medical record No: _____

Name: _____

Date of birth: _____ / _____ / _____

Gender: ☐ Male   ☐ female   Contact information: _____

Address: _____

Occupation: _____

E-mail: _____

Emergency contact: _____

Please pay attention to the following issues:

Are your eyes sensitive to various light sources?	☐ Yes / ☐ No
Does your skin get sunburned easily?	☐ Yes / ☐ No
Are you pregnant?	☐ Yes / ☐ No

Please read the content carefully:

1. Suitable candidate for professional cold light bleaching

Cold light bleaching is recommended for people who want to change the color of their teeth, but is not recommended for children under 16 and pregnant women. Depending on the cause of tooth discoloration, your doctor will make a reasonable and complete treatment plan for you.

2. Bleaching effect

Professional bleaching can be very effective, but there are many reasons for tooth discoloration and it is difficult to predict with any certainty how far your teeth will go. Yellow or yellowish brown teeth will generally bleaching faster and better than gray and grayish brown teeth. Bleaching may require more than one course of treatment for discoloration and white spots on the surface of teeth caused by antibiotics, tetracycline, root canal treatment, or trauma. During the consultation, the doctor will show you before and after the bleaching of the previous cases, so as to increase your understanding of the treatment effect of our company's tooth bleaching products. The doctor will also evaluate the possible bleaching effect of your teeth according to your dental conditions. If you have any questions, please discuss with your doctor before signing up for bleaching treatment. Each patient should complete the bleaching procedure as recommended by the doctor.

3. Maintenance

Between 24 and 48 hours after bleaching, the bleaching effect becomes more uniform and lustrous as a protective film rebuilds on the surface of the teeth. In addition, the bleaching effect will also be due to your daily eating habits as a result of the tooth re-staining process, the status of re-staining depends on the consumption of tobacco, coffee, tea, betel nut, red wine and other colored diet. These conditions can be bleached and maintained at home with self-care "home bleaching" to make the bleaching effect more lasting and stable.

4. Potential problems and risks

Any form of aesthetic treatment during operation there are varying degrees of risk and limitation, while professional teeth bleaching atractylodes rarely have problems with dangerous (If they exist, they are very small). However, we do want you to be aware of potential problems and risks. Please read the following information in detail and check with your doctor before signing if you have any questions.

(1) Sensitivity: In dental bleaching treatment, some people because there are a cracked teeth, abrasion, defect may feel a slight problems such as tooth ache. If your teeth are usually sensitive, please inform us before treatment. We will adjust the dose and the irradiation time of bleach light source to reduce your discomfort, but we cannot completely eliminate the sensitive and painful phenomenon. For some special cases of tooth sensitivity, we recommend that patients take cycoxidase inhibitors before treatment. If you feel any discomfort during the course of treatment, please inform your doctor immediately, and we will make some adjustments during the course of treatment to alleviate your discomfort. The mild soreness from bleaching usually resolves itself within 12-24 hours.

(2) Gum and oral tissue discomfort: Temporary burning may occur during the course

of treatment, usually because the oral tissue comes into contact with bleach. We will apply gum protectors for you to prevent this from happening as much as possible and completely protect your oral tissue. In addition, in order to achieve the best bleaching results, we will use a mouth opener to open your lips, so you may feel a slight discomfort, which will be resolved after the bleaching treatment. Most patients will not feel uncomfortable during treatment. If you have an uncomfortable feeling in your mouth, gargle with warm water.

(3) Resin fillings, dentures, porcelain veneers, restorations, metal crowns, etc., cannot be changed by this bleaching treatment. The results of bleaching are different from natural teeth. We will try our best to remove pigments and stains on your dentures. All restored teeth, dentures and resin fillings may be different from the color of the bleached natural teeth. Please talk to your doctor before treatment.

5. Your rights

To ensure the bleaching effect and maintain your health, please make sure that your disposable tooth bleach package is unopened before bleaching.

Authorization:

The information I have given in this document is correct.

I have read and understood the above information in detail. I have a complete understanding of the dental department and the services it provides. All my questions have been answered completely by the professionals of the institution and I am satisfied with the information and answers I have received.

Based on the above knowledge, I authorize the dental department and the professional medical staff of the institution to perform the tooth bleaching treatment and related courses for me, and AGREE to pay all the expenses.

Customer's signature: _____   Doctor's signature: _____

Date: _____   Date: _____

Chapter 6
Treatment Steps of Bleaching in the Clinic

1 Precautionary instructions and treatment of side effects

(1) No local anesthesia, patient monitoring

Local anaesthesia should not be used for bleaching. Doctors should monitor patients throughout the whole process in order to timely detect the symptoms of dental discomfort, and guide patients to raise their hands or press the alarm bell in time when any burning, tingling or discomfort occurs. If the patient develops tooth sensitivity that cannot be relieved, the treatment should be terminated immediately.

(2) Tooth sensitivity

Screening suitable patients at the initial visit and preoperative examination will minimize the possibility of tooth sensitization. Some risk factors for tooth sensitivity include decay, gum withdrawal, neck defects, or a history of tooth sensitivity.

For patients with a history of tooth sensitivity, there are three solutions: ① continuous use of toothpaste containing potassium nitrate or desensitization agent 2 weeks before surgery to relieve discomfort; ② For high-risk patients, take cyclooxygenase inhibitors or related painkillers 30 minutes before surgery; ③ During bleaching, 3%-6% potassium nitrate gel was applied to the tongue side for synchronous antisensitivity.

(3) Soft tissue burns or swelling of the lip

Gingival protectant must be carefully applied. If bleach leaks from below the gingival protectant or accidentally touches soft tissue, rinse immediately with plenty of water and apply grease, such as vitamin E or Vaseline. Grease relieves soft tissue tingling and paleness in a few hours. Vaseline or topical anesthetics can be given to patients when they return home. Antihistamines should be considered if allergic skin reactions occur.

(4) Chalk spots

As dehydration can make chalky spots more visible during bleaching treatment, as much chalky spots as possible should be found prior to treatment. Within 24 hours of treatment, these chalk spots will gradually fade as the rehydration of teeth.

(5) Light sensitive

Before using a bleach cold light machine, physicians should make sure that the patient is not taking any photosensitive medications or that the patient has a photosensitive skin condition. Adverse skin reactions may occur, with swelling of the lip and surrounding tissues.

(6) Pregnant or lactating women and minor children

We recommend delaying treatment for women who are pregnant or breast-feeding, adolescents and children.

2 Clean governance

Before bleaching, use a rubber cup or fiber brush to dip in polishing cream or pumice powder to clean the pigment and plaque on the tooth surface. (6-1 to 6-7)

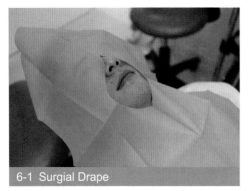
6-1 Surgial Drape

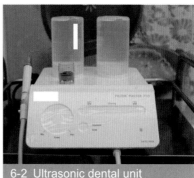
6-2 Ultrasonic dental unit

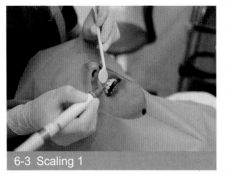
6-3 Scaling 1

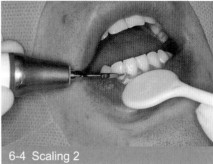
6-4 Scaling 2

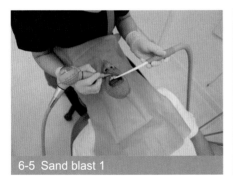

6-5 Sand blast 1

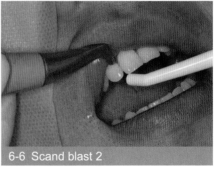

6-6 Scand blast 2

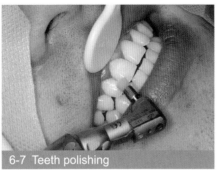

6-7 Teeth polishing

3 Preoperative colorimetry and photography

Preoperative tooth color was recorded by visual colorimetry or electronic colorimetry under natural light. Postoperative patients often forget preoperative tooth color, and preoperative colorimetric records help show improvement in tooth color after treatment. (6-8 to 6-11)

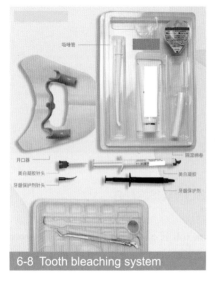

6-8 Tooth bleaching system

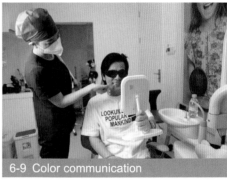

6-9 Color communication

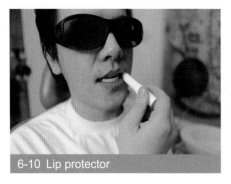

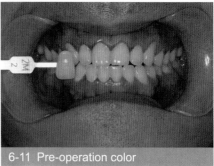

6-10 Lip protector

6-11 Pre-operation color

4 Goggles and masks

When using bleach cold light equipment, the patient must wear goggles or holes to avoid damage to the eyeball. At the same time, it is recommended to install soft cover at the light outlet to avoid harmful light scattering.

5 Lip and cheek pull and protection

Apply lipstick to the patient's lips to protect them. Vitamin E and Vaseline are fat-soluble antioxidants that neutralize accidental soft tissue damage caused by peroxides. There are a variety of lip and buccal mouth openers suitable for treatment. It is recommended to use mouth openers with tongue pads and place a towel under the mouth openers to further protect the soft tissue around the mouth. (6-12 to 6-13)

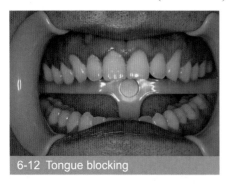

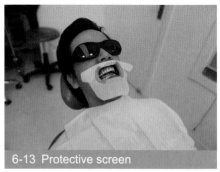

6-12 Tongue blocking

6-13 Protective screen

6 Protect the periodontal soft tissue

After the mouthpiece is in place, a damp cotton roll is placed in the vestibular groove. Dry gingival crevicular fluid and carefully apply a photocuring gum protectant along the gingival edge with a delivery tube to avoid chemical burns. The gingival protective agent can also extend 5-10mm to the root, and contact with the moist cotton roll to form a whole and seal the gingival. Use a light curing lamp that illuminates each tooth for about 10 seconds to completely cure the gum protectant. Note that photocurable lamps should be kept moving, as high power photocurable lamps may cause soft tissue discomfort. (6-14 to 6-19)

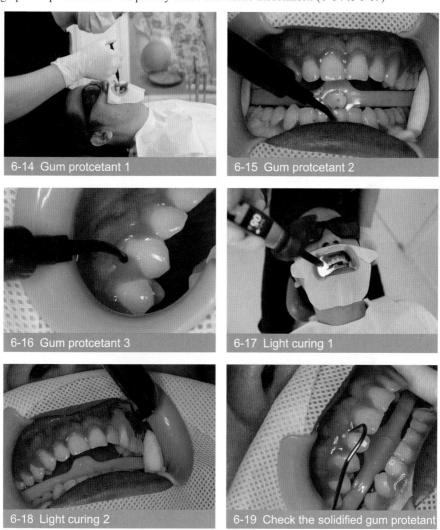

6-14 Gum protcetant 1

6-15 Gum protcetant 2

6-16 Gum protcetant 3

6-17 Light curing 1

6-18 Light curing 2

6-19 Check the solidified gum protetant

7 Activate bleach

Two-syringe mixed bleach involves mixing a syringe containing bleach with an injection containing activator and draining bubbles. Bleach stored in the refrigerator should be kept at room temperature or preheated in a hot bath.

8 Apply bleach

Apply bleach to the teeth in a thickness of 1-2mm, usually for 15-20min, and repeat twice for each visit. Prior to repeated bleach applications, old bleach should be sucked up with a surgical suction device. If the patient develops any symptoms of pain, immediately remove all bleach and rinse with plenty of water. If the insulation cotton roll is too wet, it should be replaced in time. (6-20 to 6-25)

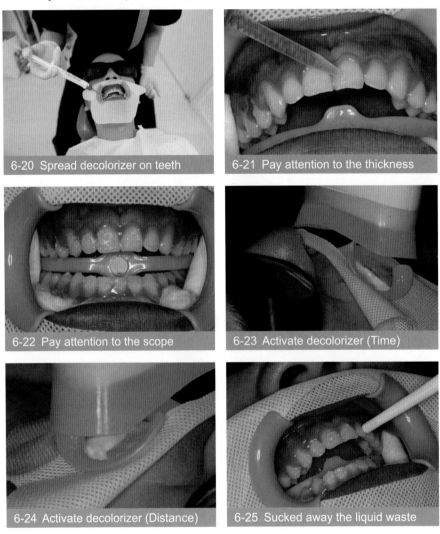

6-20 Spread decolorizer on teeth

6-21 Pay attention to the thickness

6-22 Pay attention to the scope

6-23 Activate decolorizer (Time)

6-24 Activate decolorizer (Distance)

6-25 Sucked away the liquid waste

9 Remove gum protectant

At the end of bleaching, apply a probe to remove gum protectant in one piece, taking care not to omit it.

10 Postoperative coloration

Postoperative colorimetry was performed using the same colorimetric system and documented to show immediate postoperative results. (6-26 to 6-30)

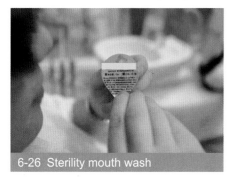

6-26 Sterility mouth wash

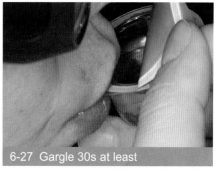

6-27 Gargle 30s at least

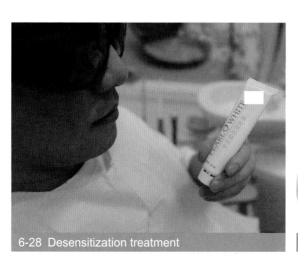

6-28 Desensitization treatment

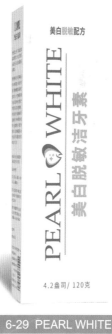

6-29 PEARL WHITE

35

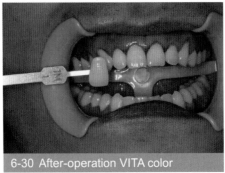
6-30 After-operation VITA color

11 Postoperative guidance

Postoperative guidelines include, but are not limited to, avoiding beverages containing pigments, such as coffee, tea and wine for at least one week. For patients who need desensitizers or painkillers before surgery, continued use after surgery can help relieve tooth sensitivity. In order to maintain the effect of bleaching, you can use home bleaching combined treatment, regular maintenance. (6-31 to 6-32)

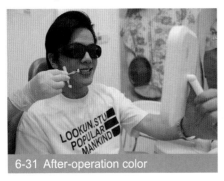
6-31 After-operation color

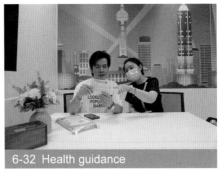
6-32 Health guidance

| Chapter 7
| Home Bleaching
| Treatment Steps

Home bleaching is a simplified treatment technique in which patients receive personalized braces or bleaching trays for home bleaching after an initial consultation with a physician. The physician gives the patient a home bleach solution with detailed instructions for use. This chapter describes in detail the techniques and methods of home bleaching to help physicians achieve successful results.

1 Precautionary instructions and treatment of side effects

Advantages and disadvantages of this technology should be clarified in detail to facilitate communication with patients:

(1) Advantages

- Simple, fast and easy to implement.
- Short chair time.
- Cost-effective.
- Low tooth sensitivity.
- High degree of freedom during treatment.

(2) Disadvantages

- Depends on the patient's cooperation.
- ·The effectiveness of bleaching depends on reaction time. If patients wear braces and bleach time does not meet the requirements, the efficacy will be reduced.
- Potential for abuse.
- Patients with high sensitivity to oral foreign bodies are difficult to cooperate.

The remaining steps include, but are not limited to, initial consultation, routine oral examination, preoperative colorimetric assessment, photography, and planning, similar to what is known as "Clinic bleaching".

2 The impression

A fine impression should be made to copy the morphology of upper and lower teeth, or the data of upper and lower teeth should be recorded by oral scanning, so as to facilitate the production of whitening trays and personalized braces. Take the mold using alginate, mixing materials, as far as possible to remove bubbles; during the mouth scan, dry the saliva with an air gun in order to get good detail.

3 Models

The production of the model is particularly important. The oral scan data can be commissioned by the denture processing center for 3D printing, and personalized braces can be made directly. Alginate impression material should be molded as soon as possible to avoid deformation. The upper and mandibular models were modified into saddle shape, and the teeth and periodontal tissues of the upper and lower jaws were preserved, excluding the jaw or lingual tissues. The model base is flat and perpendicular to the central incisors. In this way, the vacuum pressed braces are easier to fit the model and avoid the formation of various wrinkles in the process of processing.

4 Make personalized braces

Usually personalized braces will be commissioned denture processing center production, can also be made in the outpatient processing room. There is no evidence that this accelerates the bleaching process, and it is assumed that the bleaching agent degrades at the same rate with or without the bleaching agent. But the storage pool also has some advantages, such as increasing the retention of braces and reducing excessive pressure on the gums.

5 Try on braces and patient guidance

Try to wear the braces in the mouth first. If the edge of the braces is found to be more than 1mm above the covering gum, it needs to be polished smooth to avoid the stimulation of the edge of the braces on the oral soft tissue. Teach patients how to remove braces and place bleach.

6 The doctor's advice

The amount of bleach should be appropriate and should not overflow the tooth area. If there is overflow, it should be removed in time to prevent swallowing. Each wear time shall be carried out according to the product operation guide. Rinse and dry immediately after each bleaching, and store in the braces box for storage; When tooth allergy or gingival inflammation occurs, stop wearing it for 1-2 days and contact your physician. Brushing with fluoride toothpaste is recommended during bleaching.

7 Course of treatment

The total course of treatment needs to be flexibly formulated according to the actual situation, and generally needs 1-6 months. The patient is invited to return visit once every 2 weeks to understand whether the operation of the patient is correct, check the status of tooth color change, gingival inflammation, whether there is a defect of braces, etc., find the problem and solve it in time.

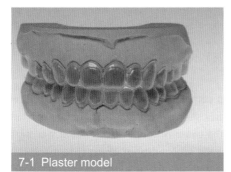
7-1 Plaster model

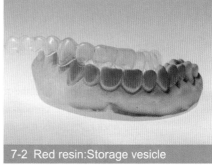
7-2 Red resin:Storage vesicle

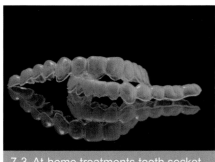
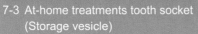
7-3 At-home treatments tooth socket (Storage vesicle)

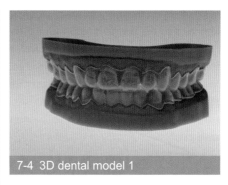
7-4 3D dental model 1

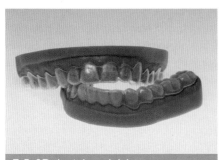
7-5 3D dental model 1

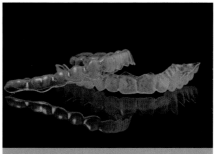
7-6 At-home treatments tooth socket (Without storage vesicle)

| Chapter 8
| Complications

1 External root resorption

External root absorption is one of the main complications of pulp-free bleaching, with an incidence of 7%. Retrospective clinical studies showed that most patients with external root absorption were under 25 years old, and the cause of tooth discoloration was mostly dental trauma. Animal studies have shown that the probability of external root resorption using thermal catalysis is 18%-25%, compared with 0%-6% without thermal catalysis. It is speculated that the mechanism of external root resorption may be that the strong oxidant penetrates into the periodontium through the dentine tubules covered by cementum (about 10% of teeth have such anatomical defects) or the defective cementum penetrates into the periodontium, causing cementum necrosis and periodontal membrane inflammation. Infection makes the inflammatory symptoms persist and finally leads to external root resorption. Such complications may be reduced by using strong sealing materials to form a protective layer, substituting weak oxidants such as sodium perborate for strong oxidants, and not using thermal catalysis.

2 Sensitive teeth

Tooth sensitivity is the main complication of extrinsic bleaching of living pulp. About 60% of patients will experience mild and transient symptoms of tooth sensitivity. However, there will be no substantial damage to the tooth pulp in general and it will be basically recovered after termination of treatment. Fluoride can be used before and after bleaching to reduce tooth sensitivity.

3 Soft tissue injury

The high concentration of hydrogen peroxide used in the clinic is easy to cause soft tissue burns, and the burn depth is usually shallow. After a large amount of water washing, anti-corrosion and anti-inflammatory drugs are applied to the wound surface, which will usually recover quickly without sequela. Soft tissue damage during home bleaching is usually caused by improper braces or trays. Normal dose of bleach will not cause obvious soft tissue damage.

4 The influence of enamel surface

Studies have shown that bleach can decrease the micro hardness of enamel surface, but bleaching with fluoride can promote remineralization. The bleaching process will release a lot of oxygen into the teeth, which inhibits the polymerization of the resin. Therefore, waiting 1-2 weeks after bleaching can reduce this side effect, which can not only achieve a good bonding effect, but also ensure a more stable color of the teeth.

5 The influence of bleaching drugs on common filling materials

(1) The influence on composite resin

Bleaching agent can increase the roughness and hardness of resin surface, but has no clinical significance; Bleaching agent contact resin material, its color does not change significantly, but will increase the resin edge microdialysis.

(2) The influence on other repair materials

Bleaching agent has no effect on porcelain and gold, and some silver amalgam can promote the release of mercury, but has no clinical significance; In addition, bleach can discolor the temporary crown of methyl methacrylate, affecting its function by altering the matrix structure in glass ionomer cement.

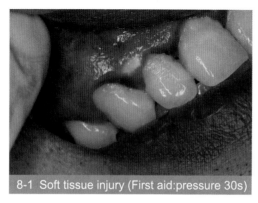

8-1 Soft tissue injury (First aid:pressure 30s)

| Chapter 9
| Special Cases

1 Tetracycline teeth

Tetracycline broad-spectrum antibiotics were introduced in 1948 and were quickly applied to treat a variety of infectious diseases in children and adults. All tetracycline compounds contain four fused rings, hence the name tetracycline. The most obvious side effect of tetracycline administration is fluorescent pigment deposition in tissues that have been mineralized at the time of administration. It can chelate calcium ions and be absorbed by teeth, cartilage and bone to form tetracycline - calcium - phosphorus complex. If used during tooth development, it can cause tooth discoloration and enamel insufficiency in deciduous permanent teeth.

(1) The aesthetic treatment of tetracycline teeth has several schemes:

- Bleaching teeth only.
- Tooth bleaching combined with composite resin filling to cover the discoloration area.
- Combined treatment: tooth bleaching and direct veneer (non-invasive veneer).
- Indirect veneer repair (invasive veneer).
- Complete crown restoration.

Different methods are suitable for different degrees of tetracycline teeth. In principle, invasive and minimally invasive treatment should be the first choice. This chapter mainly discusses the problems of tooth bleaching.

(2) The degree of tetracycline tooth discoloration is classified and suggestions are given:

- Grade I: mild tetracycline teeth. Yellow to gray uniform discoloration, no strip change.
- Grade II: moderate tetracycline teeth. Brown to dark gray discoloration.
- Grade III: severe tetracycline teeth. Bluish gray or black discoloration with distinct bands.
- Grade IV: difficult cases, bleaching is usually ineffective.
- Grade V: severe discoloration, quality defect, not an indication.

In general, degree I-III tetracycline bleaching is effective. The best option is to start bleaching first and then evaluate the need for more invasive treatment.

(3) Tetracycline tooth bleaching treatment is as follows:

- Long-term family bleaching, long-term effect is good.
- Home bleaching and clinic bleaching combined treatment.
- Internal bleaching after intentional root canal treatment. But this approach is so radical and controversial that it is hardly recommended today.

2　Dental fluorosis

Dental fluorosis is a prominent symptom of regional chronic fluorosis. Regional chronic fluorosis is an endemic disease that mainly affects the bones and developing teeth. Severe chronic fluorosis with bone lesions, known as skeletal fluorosis; the chronic fluorosis with only dental lesions is called dental fluorosis. Dental fluorosis is a special type of enamel hypoplasia. It is also called dental fluorosis or enamel enamel because the affected teeth mainly show colored plaque and defect on enamel clinically.

Dental fluorosis is an endemic disease and the concentrated distribution of dental fluorosis is called the endemic area of dental fluorosis. Dean classification is commonly used in clinical and epidemiological investigations of dental fluorosis, which was the earliest classification survey for dental fluorosis proposed in 1942 and is also the classification standard recommended by the World Health Organization:

- Normal: The enamel surface is smooth and shiny, usually milky white.
- Suspicious: Slight changes in the opacity of the enamel, from a few white markings to occasional white spots.
- Very light: Small papery white opaque areas irregularly distributed over the tooth surface, but not exceeding 25% of the tooth surface.
- Mild: The white opaque area on the tooth surface is more extensive, but does not exceed 50% of the tooth surface.
- Moderate: There is significant wear on the enamel surface, and it is tan or tan.
- Severe: The enamel surface is seriously involved, with obvious hypoplasia and extensive brown staining, which affects the appearance of the whole tooth.

In general, mild teeth without significant defects can be treated with bleaching or a combination of microgrinding and osmotic resin. Ceramic restorations are recommended for moderate and severe tooth defects.

3　Nonvital teeth

Nonvital tooth bleaching technology is mainly used to improve the discoloration of teeth caused by trauma or pulp treatment. Although all-porcelain/zirconium crown restoration is commonly used in clinical treatment of non-medullary teeth, there are still some cases that need bleaching treatment. The clinical efficacy of this method is not lasting, the color recovery rate is 83%-91%, 1-5 years after treatment, 50%-65% of affected teeth can show different degrees of color regression. This chapter mainly introduces the crown bleaching method:

Intra coronal bleaching is a common method of nonvital tooth bleaching. It uses a high concentration of bleach and must be performed in the clinic. There are two methods: thermocatalytic bleaching and progressive bleaching. The thermocatalytic process involves heating 22%-35% of the hydrogen peroxide into the medullary cavity several times over a 30-minute period, followed by a thorough flushing. Thermal catalysis has the advantages of high efficacy and short course of treatment, but its disadvantage is that it is easy to cause external absorption of tooth root. The progressive bleaching method has a shorter and safer time per visit, but the course of treatment is relatively long.

Progressive bleaching is a common clinical technique, and the steps are as follows:

- Perfect root canal therapy. Before bleaching, X-rays must be taken to confirm that the canal has been properly filled.
- Install rubber barriers to protect the gums from being burned by strong oxidants.
- Medullary cavity cleaning. The slow speed ball drill removes the contents of the pulp cavity and uncovers the top of the pulp to ensure that the pulp Angle and other areas that may conceal pulp tissue are fully exposed. If there is a resin filling in the pulp cavity, clean it carefully. Do not leave any resin material, so that the bleach can contact closely with the dentin and penetrate effectively.
- Remove part of the root filling, with zinc phosphate cement or glass ion cement and other materials at the bottom, to form a protective layer, prevent the infiltration of bleach to the root. The thickness of the base material should be at least 2mm, and the height of the crown should be in line with the attachment epithelium of the gingiva, so that the bleach can penetrate the "S" shaped dentin tubules in the neck of the tooth and remove the crown color.
- Place bleach. A high concentration of hydrogen peroxide solution is placed directly into the medullary cavity. For safety, sodium perborate and water/saline can also be mixed into a paste or 10% urea peroxide into the medullary cavity.
- The medullary cavity was closed. Use viscous sealer to block bleach agent, such as glass ion or resin, to avoid bleach leakage.
- Follow-up visit. Determine the interval between follow-up visits depending on the bleaching agent used. Tooth color should be recorded at each follow-up visit. The number of visits depends on the change of color, and usually 3-6 visits are required. After bleaching, the color of the teeth should be slightly whiter than that of the teeth of the same maxillary name to leave room for the color to recede. If the desired goal is not reached after repeated visits, and the color has no significant change, the patient's opinion should be sought, bleaching treatment should be terminated, and repair treatment should be performed according to the needs.
- Completion. Two weeks after the end of bleaching treatment, the pulp cavity was filled with a suitable dental-colored composite resin.

Chapter 10
Postoperative
Management

In the previous chapters, we have emphasized the importance of preoperative communication and standardized treatment plan, and postoperative management is mainly carried out around this central idea, mainly involving three aspects: the persistence of treatment, side effects after treatment and safety issues.

1 Persistence

This topic is the most concerned issue for patients. Although many literatures and propaganda emphasize the "persistence" and "satisfaction" of bleaching treatment, the persistence of bleaching cannot be "mythic" because of the different evaluation standards of various experts and scholars.

The first question is "How long will the bleaching effect last?" Objective cognition started from the literature. In 1990, Dr. Van Haywood followed up the patient cohort for 12 years: 74% were satisfied with color 1.5 years after surgery, and the satisfaction rate decreased to 62% 3 years after surgery. In 2002, Ritter followed up the patient cohort for 9-12 years. Results: The average color retention rate and satisfaction rate were 43% after 10 years of treatment. In a 2011 Leonard follow-up report of 47 months, whitening was maintained in 89% of patients, and 82% of patients had improved tooth color by at least 2 color scales from baseline, with an average color improvement by 5 Vita palette units.

The second question is "Whether bleaching again is required and, if so, how often?" The 1994 Haywood study reported that bleaching again was required on average 25 months after treatment. In 2011, Leonard reported that whitening occurred again in the 32nd month.

Another core factor is the postoperative diet structure of patients. Different guidelines have different answers for the immediate postoperative diet, mainly focusing on not drinking any colored drinks at least 6 hours to 2 weeks after surgery, which is quite controversial.

To sum up,our suggestions are as follows: ① the duration of color maintenance after bleaching treatment is 1.5-2 years; ② the maximum frequency of bleaching again, i.e. polishing bleaching, is 7 days; ③ do not drink any colored beverages for at least 48-72 hours after bleaching.

2 Post-treatment side effects

As mentioned in the previous chapter, the main side effects after bleaching are gingival irritation and tooth sensitivity.

(1) Gingival irritation mainly occurs during home bleaching.

The most likely reason is that the tray edge extends to the gum and bleach is retained at the gum edge. You can solve this problem by trimming the edges of your braces. Note that even if the braces do not completely cover the entire surface of the tooth, the teeth can turn white as time passes and bleach penetrates and moves between the glaze columns.

(2) There are many reasons for tooth sensitivity.

First of all, problems caused by non-standard intraoperative operation or excessive dehydration should be excluded. The second consideration is the degree of hardness and adhesion of braces, whether the "orthodontic force" is generated, and the third evaluation is the choice of household bleach concentration, whether the increased risk of sensitivity. It is recommended to use toothpaste containing potassium nitrate and fluoride for 2 weeks at home before surgery. 3% potassium nitrate and 0.11% fluoride desensitization agent were used for more than 30 minutes before surgery. Use desensitization agents consistently during home bleaching.

At the same time, doctors should emphasize to patients the importance of postoperative diet structure, control lemon acidic fruit, juice, cola and other carbonated drinks and areca nut hard food.

3 Security issues

After tooth bleaching, patients do not often experience side effects such as caries rate, tooth breakage, oral pathological changes or pulp pathological changes. In general, the only long-term change after bleaching is a lighter tooth color than immediately after bleaching. Bleaching is as effective and safe as any other standard dental treatment.

Main References

［1］樊明文，周学东. 牙体牙髓病学［M］. 北京：人民卫生出版社，2016.

［2］高学军，岳林. 牙体牙髓病学［M］. 北京：北京大学出版社，2017.

［3］Linda Greenwall，刘擎，周锐（译）. 牙齿美白 Tooth Whitening Techniques

　　［M］. 沈阳：辽宁科技出版社，2020.

牙齿漂白
临床实用手册
（中英对照）

Clinical Operation Techniques of
Tooth Bleaching

孟 超 沈 健 况小明 主 编

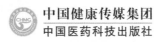

中国健康传媒集团

中国医药科技出版社

内 容 提 要

　　本书就牙齿漂白术的临床操作技术进行了系统的阐述，以图解的形式直观地诠释了牙齿漂白术的规范化操作，书中经验多来自多年临床一线的病例累积，借此书为临床医师正确、规范地开展和看待此技术提供指导和帮助。

图书在版编目（CIP）数据

　　牙齿漂白临床实用手册 = Clinical Operation Techniques of Tooth Bleaching：汉英对照 / 孟超，沈健，况小明主编 . — 北京：中国医药科技出版社，2022.11
　　ISBN 978-7-5214-3392-0

　　Ⅰ . ①牙…　Ⅱ . ①孟…　②沈…　③况…　　Ⅲ . ①牙—美容术—手册—汉、英　Ⅳ . ① R783

　　中国版本图书馆 CIP 数据核字（2021）第 164417 号

责任编辑　　张芳芳　　郭紫薇
美术编辑　　陈君杞
版式设计　　也　在

出版　**中国健康传媒集团** | 中国医药科技出版社
地址　北京市海淀区文慧园北路甲 22 号
邮编　100082
电话　发行：010-62227427　　邮购：010-62236938
网址　www.cmstp.com
规格　710 × 1000 mm $^1/_{16}$
印张　6 $^3/_4$
字数　122 千字
版次　2022 年 11 月第 1 版
印次　2022 年 11 月第 1 次印刷
印刷　北京盛通印刷股份有限公司
经销　全国各地新华书店
书号　ISBN 978-7-5214-3392-0
定价　**35.00 元**

获取新书信息、投稿、为图书纠错，请扫码联系我们。

编委会

前言

　　随着社会的不断发展，医学技术及医学理念也在不断更新，大众对牙齿的美观要求越来越高，牙齿变色成为一个必须要解决的问题。越来越多的患者要求漂白牙齿，改善牙齿颜色。尽管在全瓷修复技术风靡的当下，改善牙齿颜色可以有更多的治疗手段，但是其带来的创伤是不可逆转和不可忽视的。患者和医师都谋求无创的治疗技术，这就使得牙齿漂白术再次得到重视，使用次数增加。

　　现代科学技术的发展使牙齿漂白技术和理念不断更新，不同浓度的漂白剂、脱敏剂、电子比色仪、冷光漂白仪的应用使牙齿漂白术成功率增加。高成功率的牙齿漂白技术有助于临床医师更好地治疗变色牙齿。

　　本书就牙齿漂白术的临床操作技术进行了系统的阐述，希望为临床医师更广泛地开展此技术提供指导和帮助。

孟　超

2022 年 5 月

目录

绪论

　　牙齿漂白术已经有将近 145 年的历史，是一项基础且已经非常普及的临床实用技术。我们应当正视该技术，既不能"神话"也不能"轻视"。从适应证的角度来说，可应用牙齿漂白术的实际比例是相当大的。因此，作为口腔执业医师应当了解并规范掌握该技术。

　　编者累积了大量的临床经验和知识，同时聘请了 12 位在该领域有丰富经验的医师和学者作为顾问，通过此书系统地阐述了牙齿漂白术的过程和注意事项。书中经验来自多年临床一线的病例累积，借此书为同行们如何正确规范地开展和看待该技术提供帮助。

　　《牙齿漂白临床实用手册》以图解形式直观地诠释了牙齿漂白术的规范化操作，相信它能在帮助临床医师进行牙齿变色治疗方面发挥积极作用。

第一章
牙齿变色

正常牙齿是有光泽的黄白色，因身体和（或）牙齿内部发生改变所致的牙齿色泽的变化称为牙齿变色，又称内源性牙齿着色。进入口腔的外来色素或口腔中细菌携带或产生的色素在牙齿表面沉积导致的牙齿着色称之为外源性牙齿着色。

牙齿变色包括由局部因素造成的个别牙齿变色和全身因素引起的多颗牙或全口牙齿变色，例如四环素牙、氟斑牙等。

外源性牙齿着色是指牙齿外表着色，与生活习惯有关，例如食物、饮料或烟草均可引起牙齿着色；某些药物所携带的成分也可以引起着色，例如氟化亚锡、氯己定等。随着年龄的变化，牙齿对外源性着色的敏感性也会不断提高。外源性着色经常与牙齿表面的唾液蛋白膜、牙菌斑或牙结石共同存在。

一　变色的原因

牙齿变色是复杂的物理和化学过程，有色物质与牙齿组织在生理或病理状态下的结合均会导致牙齿的变色，有关原因如下。

1. 牙髓出血

牙齿外伤或使用砷剂失活牙髓时导致牙髓血管破裂，或因机械拔髓时出血过多，血液分解的产物渗入牙本质小管，使周围牙本质变色。变色的程度随时间延长而加重。外伤所致的牙髓出血在早期使牙冠呈现粉红色，随血液渗入髓腔壁到达牙本质层，后期牙冠会呈现浅灰色、浅棕或灰棕色。

2. 牙髓坏死

坏死的牙髓会产生硫化氢，与血红蛋白发生反应后形成黑色的硫化铁。黑色素也可来自产黑色素的病原菌。黑色物质缓慢渗入牙本质小管，使牙齿呈灰黑色或黑色。

3. 牙本质过度钙化

外伤后，牙齿髓腔内沿根管壁过度形成不规则牙本质，造成牙冠部透明度降低，使牙齿表现为黄色或黄棕色。

4. 饮食因素

食物、饮料、槟榔和烟草有累积的变色效果。尤其是有釉质和牙本质裂纹、磨损现象的中老年人更为明显。

5. 牙本质脱水

无髓牙失去了来自牙髓的营养支持，牙本质脱水致使牙齿表面失去原有的半透明光泽，呈现晦暗的灰色。

6. 医源性因素

（1）残髓：根管治疗过程中残留的牙髓逐渐分解导致牙齿变色。

（2）窝洞和根管内用的药物或充填材料：例如碘化物、金霉素等可使牙齿变为浅黄色、浅褐色或浅灰色；银汞合金和铜汞合金可使充填体周围的牙齿变成黑色；酚醛树脂可使牙齿呈红棕色等。

二　变色的分类

健康的天然牙齿颜色并不是均匀一致的，由于牙釉质和牙本质的厚度、对光的反射以及透明度的不同，牙齿颈部、体部和切端的颜色是逐渐变化的。

由于不同的牙齿变色对漂白治疗的敏感性不同，只有仔细评估牙齿变色的类型和诱因才能制定完善的漂白治疗计划，获得良好的漂白效果。

牙齿变色可分为外源性变色和内源性变色两种类型。

1. 外源性变色——着色物质影响了牙釉质表面

（1）生活习惯：如长期喝茶、喝咖啡、吸食烟草制品或嚼槟榔的人，牙齿表面，特别是舌面有褐色或黑褐色着色，刷牙不能去除；牙齿的窝沟和表面粗糙处也易着色。

（2）口腔卫生不良：外来色素首先沉着于牙面的黏液膜和菌斑中。口腔卫生不良者，菌斑滞留处，如近龈缘处、邻接面是经常着色的部位。随着菌斑下方牙齿表面的脱矿，色素也可渗入牙体组织内部。

（3）药物因素：长期使用氯己定、高锰酸钾溶液漱口或用药物牙膏，例如氯己定牙膏可在牙齿表面形成浅褐色或深褐色着色；牙齿局部使用氨制硝酸银处理后，相应部位会变成黑色。

（4）职业性接触：因工作需要接触某些矿物，如铁、硫等，牙齿可着褐色；接触铜、镍、铬等，牙齿表面可出现绿色沉着物。

（5）其他因素：唾液的黏稠度、酸碱度以及口腔内携产色素细菌的生长均与外来色素沉积有关；年龄的变化也会使牙齿对外源性着色的敏感性不断提高。

2. 内源性变色——牙齿结构的变色

（1）病因来源于牙齿萌出前：例如血液疾病，牙釉质或牙本质发育不良等。

（2）病因来源于牙齿发育期间：例如服用四环素，摄入氟过量等。

（3）病因来源于牙齿萌出后：例如各种因素造成的牙髓坏死、牙外伤、龋齿，修复材料和牙科某些操作步骤，以及一些牙齿的增龄性变化（釉质变薄，继发性牙本质增加等）。

第二章
牙齿漂白技术

　　牙齿漂白技术是通过使用化学物质氧化牙齿中的有机色素而使牙齿颜色变浅的方法。与其他改善牙齿颜色的美学技术相比，漂白治疗的优点是在治疗过程中对患牙创伤小，可最大限度地保持牙齿硬组织的完整性，且临床操作技术简单；缺点是治疗时间稍长，远期漂白效果持续时间不易预测，部分病例的预后可能达不到患者的预期值，治疗前应向患者说明。

一　化学反应

　　漂白剂一般为氧化剂，与变色牙体组织发生氧化还原反应。漂白剂置于牙齿后，可释放活性氧；过氧化物弥散进入牙本质结构内，到达管周牙本质，这一过程伴随氧化反应的发生。通过化学反应，变色物质总量减少，转变为无色物质。

　　釉质可看作一层半透明膜的结构，漂白剂可穿透釉质进入牙齿内，其表面积很重要。漂白剂发挥活性主要依靠复杂的氧化反应，释放出氧及其他自由基；氧和其他自由基通过釉柱间的空隙结构穿透到牙本质内，从而实现漂白牙齿的作用。

　　漂白剂在放置后 5~10 分钟内即可从釉质渗透到牙本质及牙髓。同时漂白剂易从牙齿最薄弱的位置渗透，例如裂纹、裂理面、脱矿区域或白垩斑等矿化不良的区域。

　　漂白是一项非常复杂的过程，受多种因素影响，包括：①漂白剂的 pH；②漂白剂的使用方式和时间；③光照的变化；④光照的时间；⑤光线波长的选择性吸收；⑥牙齿的结构。

二 治疗对象

根据治疗对象的不同，牙齿漂白可分为活髓牙漂白和无髓牙漂白，分别包括诊室漂白和家庭漂白两种方式。顾名思义，诊室漂白是由医师在诊室内完成漂白治疗；家庭漂白是患者离开诊室后，在家使用低浓度漂白剂漂白牙齿。

无论是诊室漂白还是家庭漂白，都需要在术前正确判断牙齿变色的原因，了解患者的期望值，与患者就疗程、费用、预期效果及可能的并发症等进行充分沟通，选择并制定最佳的治疗方案，取得患者的密切配合。在进行漂白治疗时，对牙齿颜色的记录非常重要，首先用比色板或电子比色仪确定患者漂白前的牙齿颜色作为基线值，在患者见证下记录在案，漂白治疗后再次用同样比色手段确定牙齿颜色并记录。还可以为患者拍摄牙齿近距离照片和微笑照片作为补充记录，所有照片应在同样的环境、体位和放大条件下拍摄，通过比较漂白前后的牙齿颜色评估漂白效果。

三 影响因素

1. 牙齿表面清洁

在漂白前彻底清洁牙齿表面，保证漂白剂与牙齿表面充分接触。一般建议在牙齿洁治后 2 周开始漂白治疗，以减少洁治带来的牙齿敏感和牙龈问题。

2. 过氧化物浓度

随着过氧化物的浓度增高，氧化作用增强，漂白速度会加快。使用高浓度过氧化氢时，要注意保护牙龈，避免化学灼伤。

3. 温度

温度越高，氧释放的速度越快，牙齿颜色改变的速度也越快。当温度升高到令人不适的水平时，会引起牙齿敏感甚至不可复性的牙髓炎症。

4. pH

过氧化氢在酸性 pH 条件下有助于在运输和储存过程中保持它的效力。而在漂白过程中，过氧化氢发挥效果最佳的 pH 为 9.5~10.8。

5. 时间

漂白的效果直接与漂白剂和牙面接触的时间相关。在一定范围内，接触时间越长，漂白效果越好，但同时患者术后牙齿敏感的可能性也会增加。

6. 漂白剂的储存环境

将过氧化氢置于密闭的环境中可以维持它的漂白效力。

第三章
牙齿漂白的材料和设备

 漂白剂

漂白剂一般为氧化剂，常用的漂白剂有各种浓度的过氧化氢、过硼酸钠和过氧化脲。

1.过氧化氢

过氧化氢是最有效的漂白剂，各种浓度（3%~40%）均可使用，主要用于冠外漂白，也可用于冠内漂白。但高浓度的过氧化氢对软组织有腐蚀性，接触后会有剧烈的烧灼感，临床使用时应注意防护。高浓度过氧化氢受热易分解，应避光冷藏保存。

2.过氧化脲

过氧化脲相对稳定，分解后可产生脲、氨气、二氧化碳和过氧化氢，10% 的过氧化脲分解后可产生近 3.5% 的过氧化氢。常用浓度为 5%~20%，对牙髓及周围组织有刺激，主要用于冠外漂白。

3.过硼酸钠

过硼酸钠是一种氧化剂，可制成各种剂型。新鲜的过硼酸钠含有 95% 的过硼酸盐，可释放 9.9% 的氧气；干燥的过硼酸钠比较稳定，当遇到酸、热或水时可分解成偏硼酸钠、水及生态氧。

二　常用器械

1. 检查器械

检查器械包括口镜、镊子、普通探针、牙周探针、弱吸管、三用枪管、患者保护眼镜、洞巾、漱口杯。（图 3-1~ 图 3-4）

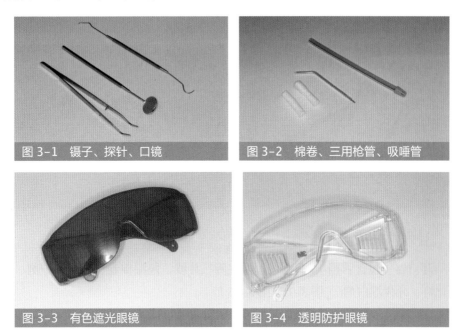

图 3-1　镊子、探针、口镜

图 3-2　棉卷、三用枪管、吸唾管

图 3-3　有色遮光眼镜

图 3-4　透明防护眼镜

2. 术前器械

印模托盘 / 口腔扫描保护套、超声波洁牙机（包括母机和工作尖）、喷砂机、低速抛光机（包括橡皮杯和抛光膏 / 浮石粉）、比色系统（比色板 / 电子比色仪）。（图 3-5~ 图 3-10）

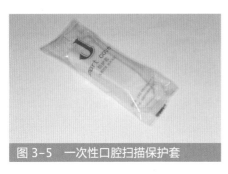

图 3-5　一次性口腔扫描保护套

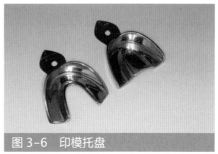

图 3-6　印模托盘

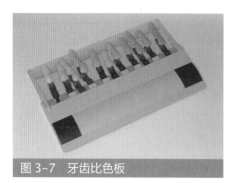

图 3-7　牙齿比色板

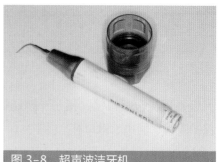

图 3-8　超声波洁牙机

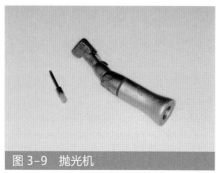

图 3-9　抛光机

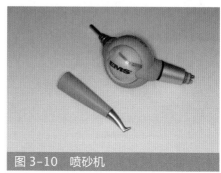

图 3-10　喷砂机

3. 术中器械

开口器（包含舌挡）、润唇膏、橡皮障、牙线、隔湿棉卷、牙龈保护剂、光固化灯、牙齿漂白剂。（图 3-11~ 图 3-16）

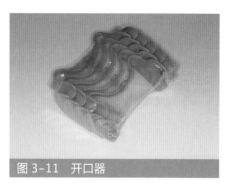

图 3-11　开口器

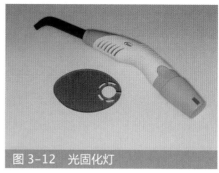

图 3-12　光固化灯

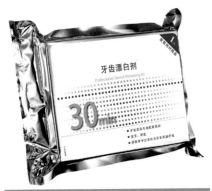

图 3-13　牙齿漂白套装（单人装）

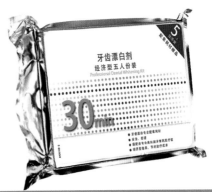

图 3-14　牙齿漂白套装（五人装）

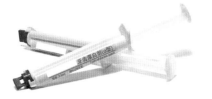

图 3-15　牙齿漂白剂

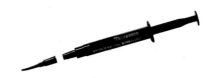

图 3-16　牙龈保护剂

三　常用设备

（1）牙齿漂白仪。

（2）电子比色仪。

（3）口腔扫描仪。

（4）光固化灯。

（5）超声波洁牙机。

（6）喷砂机。

第四章
病例选择

 适应证

牙齿漂白术适应证比较广泛，主要分为活髓牙、无髓牙和特殊病例。

1. 活髓牙漂白适应证

（1）外源性变色：是临床上最主要的病例，主要来源于饮食结构，例如茶叶、咖啡、槟榔、烟草制品和染色调味品；还来源于药物染色，例如长期使用氯己定或高锰酸钾漱口水和牙膏造成的染色。

（2）牙本质过度钙化。

（3）年龄增长导致的牙齿对外源性着色的敏感性不断提高。

（4）口腔卫生不良。

（5）职业性接触：因工作需要接触某些矿物而导致的牙齿染色。

2. 无髓牙漂白适应证

（1）牙髓出血。

（2）牙本质脱水。

3. 特殊病例

（1）遗传性釉质发育不全（白垩斑、白纹等白色病损）：有一些患者牙釉质的质地可能呈白垩样，甚至干酪样的致密度，或较坚硬。对于该类牙齿通常首先进行漂白治疗，若术后白垩斑淡化，则无须再接受其他治疗；若效果不理想，则需要结合微研磨技术或牙体修复技术恢复外形和色彩。

（2）营养缺乏、发热性疾病和低钙血症引起的釉质发育缺陷：牙釉质表面凹陷，凹陷处容易着色。对于该类牙齿通常首先进行漂白治疗，若术后着色处淡化，则无需再接受其他治疗。

（3）氟牙症：着色较轻或着色较深而无明显缺损的患牙可用漂白脱色法脱色；但重度有缺损的患牙需复合树脂、烤瓷、玻璃陶瓷贴面或全冠等方法修复。

（4）四环素牙：四环素牙是变色牙中特殊的一类，它的染色区域是牙本质，漂白剂不易透过牙釉质到达染色区，因此治疗难度大。淡黄色的变色病例及变色区域局限在切端的病例治疗效果好，较重的灰黑色预后较差，但大多数会有所改善，80% 的病例可保持 1 年以上的疗效。对四环素牙明显有效的脱色方法是冠内漂白法，即将牙髓摘除、根管充填，利用无髓牙漂白技术，使药物直接作用于变色的牙本质。该方法虽然效果明显，但副作用同样明显，临床慎用。中度染色或釉质严重缺损的牙可做烤瓷、玻璃陶瓷贴面或全冠修复，也可以先脱色，后遮盖性修复（但随着遮色剂的进步，该步骤未来或许会被淘汰）。

二　禁忌证

牙齿漂白术的绝对禁忌证很少，多数禁忌证是相对的，通常与解剖条件、口腔健康程度和患者预期有关。

1. 解剖条件

（1）乳牙 / 混合牙列。

（2）牙隐裂或髓腔过大。

（3）釉质发育不全。

（4）牙齿局部变色可通过充填修复体手段改善者。

（5）因局部解剖条件，手术视野及手术器械使用受限：例如开口受限，无法有效暴露足够口腔视野进行操作；另外由于视野及器械入路的限制，例如开口器和舌挡难以稳定，往往使一个常规的牙齿漂白术变得难以实施。

2. 口腔健康

（1）牙本质过敏症患者。

（2）牙周病变。

（3）牙齿有大面积充填物和修复体。

（4）孕妇、哺乳期妇女和化学物质过敏者。

3. 患者预期

当患者对牙齿漂白术缺乏正确认知，包括对颜色有过高的要求，对远期效果有苛刻的保障要求，欲将漂白术和修复体进行对比等，需要仔细评估和把握手术风险。有心理障碍的患者，必要时需请专科医师会诊，给予适当治疗，待疾病平稳后择期手术。

第五章
治疗计划

治疗计划的制定是漂白治疗必不可少的一步，因为漂白治疗通常是一系列美学治疗的起始。口腔执业医师需要为患者制定一套详尽的治疗方案，应当仔细认真地制定治疗计划，向患者全面地解释牙齿漂白治疗的原理、漂白治疗前应完成的必要前期治疗和漂白治疗后所涉及到的注意事项。改善并保持口腔健康是制定治疗计划的首要考虑因素。

在评估患者前，医师应理解患者在口腔健康方面的需求和要求。可以询问一位新患者"您最想要解决什么问题？""您对自己的牙齿有什么期望？"患者可能有自己的特殊想法和具体担心之处，希望与医师进行讨论和沟通。尽管部分患者以往没有仔细考虑过，也有部分患者有自己的牙科"治疗计划书"，包含了自己希望改善的地方，会有明确的美学改善需求。

本章节列举了制定牙齿漂白完善治疗计划所要求的各方面，描述了如何执行漂白治疗计划，展示了收集信息的方法，强调了全身病史和牙科既往史的重要性，讨论了患者沟通、微笑分析、患者预期、知情同意书等。本章节提供了实用问卷和表格模板，可用于信息收集阶段。

一 医患沟通

在进行任何的牙科治疗前，均应与患者建立良好明确的沟通。医师必须明确患者的需求，准确理解患者对自己牙齿变色的担忧之处，以及相应的美学需求。美是一种抽象的主观概念，但也是人性中必不可少的一部分。文化、年龄、性别、职业及时间等均影响患者对美的理解。考虑到这种主观性，在治疗初期医患之间就应建立良好的沟通，共同向一个目标努力。良好的沟通可提高治疗接受度。为做到知情同意，患者需了解治疗的益处、风险、优势和缺陷，以及拒绝治疗会带来的问题和每种治疗方式的重要性。医师应在治疗开始前与患者沟通治疗风险与益处。当患者的预期超出实际时，良好的沟通尤其重要。

医师可使用调查问卷评估患者对自己微笑的期望，问卷包括患者对自己牙齿和微笑的自我感知。问题应为开放式，允许患者表达自己的任何担心之处；还可以询问患者关于牙齿形态、位置、颜色和比例等问题。收集的信息能够确定出一个基准线，医师可依据这一基线与患者互动、沟通，评估患者的美学需求。

值得强调的是，医师应询问患者的期望值和对最终治疗结果的认知。漂白治疗前必须从全面的牙齿和口腔健康评估开始，使用清单收集信息有助于获得所有必要的信息。

二 方案设计和知情同意

1. 新患者清单

每位新患者在咨询阶段，都应收集以下信息：

（1）接受检查的知情同意。

（2）全身病史。

（3）既往牙科治疗史。

（4）口外检查。

（5）口内检查：软组织检查、牙列检查、牙周检查、咬合检查、颞下颌关节功能、牙髓活力。

（6）数码 X 光景片。

（7）其他信息：研究模型 / 口扫电子模型、口内相机照片。

2. 全身病史

医师应仔细评估患者全身情况。既往慢性病史或长期应用抗生素（四环素等）可能导致牙齿变色；早产儿可能出现釉质发育不良或牙齿出现白垩斑和白色病损。医师应让患者填写漂白专用问卷，评估患者的饮食结构：吸烟习惯、饮食习惯、是否咀嚼槟榔等。患者应当在漂白期间改变饮食结构和生活习惯，例如戒烟或减少吸烟量。

医师应注意患者是否对塑料、过氧化物或其他漂白系统内含有的成分过敏；应在全身病史页记录患者目前的用药情况，尤其是可能导致口干的药物，如抗组胺药物。服用激素的患者偶尔可出现牙龈水肿过度。目前没有关于漂白治疗对发育中胚胎影响的研究，故孕期患者和哺乳期患者不应接受漂白治疗。

3. 牙科治疗史

医师应分析牙齿变色的原因，不同原因（如龋齿、内吸收、外吸收、外伤、药物等）需要不同的治疗方法。

外源性着色通常可以通过完善的牙科专业洁治（超声波洁治、喷砂、低速抛光）去除。

4. 微笑分析和美学

什么是美丽的微笑？其中一个定义是：牙齿的大小、位置和颜色相互协调，牙齿之间互相对称成比例，且与周围组织协调。牙齿仅仅是微笑美学的一部分，要在牙龈软组织、牙弓内颊廊区和唇以及面部等组成的框架内观察。

牙齿漂白可能无法满足患者的所有需求。漂白治疗前应对患者进行微笑分析，该项目应包括在治疗计划阶段。微笑分析表可用于确定患者对微笑的要求。进行微笑分析时需要考虑许多因素：牙齿的形态和长度、唇线、笑线及牙齿咬合关系，每种因素都是一项重要的特征，所有这些特征交织在一起，就可以共同达到美学的和谐。

5. 口内检查

医师应在漂白治疗前检查患者的牙齿和牙周情况，记录下不良修复体，与患者讨论。主要评估以下方面。

（1）釉质厚度。

（2）牙龈高度或牙龈退缩量。

（3）牙齿敏感程度：牙本质敏感症和隐裂。

（4）牙齿通透度。

（5）白垩斑或白色病损：治疗后不会消失且有可能短期内加重。

（6）条带状变色：因四环素牙或脱水造成，治疗后依然会呈条带状，需术前告知。

（7）牙龈炎：需要先治疗牙龈炎或牙周炎。

（8）脱水线：年龄增长会导致釉质变薄，第三期牙本质沉积导致牙本质增厚和牙齿增龄性变黄。因该过程不均匀会产生脱水线，同时也无法均匀变白，会沿脱水线呈现出 2 个色调。

（9）暗色裂纹和病损：通常由吸烟、槟榔和夜间磨牙导致。

6. 特殊检查

（1）牙髓活力测试：可采用冷热温度测试或电活力测试。

（2）影像学检查：原则上所有漂白治疗前均应拍摄根尖片。最好拍摄全景片筛查是否有病理性问题、龋齿、根尖炎症等；特殊疾病处应辅助 CBCT 排查。漂白治疗可能诱发根尖周病变急性发作，单颗牙的变色有可能是因为死髓，此类问题均应术前确认和排查。

（3）口内数码照：可记录术前状态，对分析龋齿、裂纹、缺损、修复体和牙齿状态有很大的帮助。

（4）诊断模型：因为可能开展家庭漂白治疗，需要牙列模型制作个性化牙套。常规方法为印模后灌制石膏和口扫数据 3D 打印。

7. 美学区有旧修复体

医师必须事先告知患者，虽然旧修复体颜色与牙齿匹配，但漂白治疗后牙齿颜色变浅，可能需要更换旧修复体以更好地匹配颜色。复合树脂充填体不会因漂白而改变颜色，但有时漂白治疗会将旧修复体边缘的变色部分去除，使旧修复体看起来颜色变浅。另外，漂白治疗还会降低釉质对粘接治疗的敏感性。

8. 患者预期

在进行任何漂白治疗前，医师必须评估患者的期望。追求"纯白色牙齿""好莱坞白""明星牙"的患者很少会对牙齿漂白治疗的效果满意。医师可以在治疗前用比色板向患者讲解色号的变化。患者应该知晓，一些牙齿可能无法漂白，一些牙齿可能无法均匀变白；牙齿颜色越暗，漂白所需时间越长；老年患者靠近根面的漂白效果差，所需漂白时间长；不同年龄段患者治疗时间和预约安排不同。在漂白治疗前，医师应事先告知患者这些内容，同时应该告诉患者靠近根部和牙颈部的风险。

9. 漂白治疗照片拍摄

医师必须遵照标准流程拍摄照片，以供制定治疗计划。照片质量要高，要标准化，有条件的应使用单反相机，拍摄术前术后对比照片；数码照片可裁剪，易于标准化，便于建立术前术后对比照片病例库。

患者常常忘记治疗前牙齿的颜色和变色情况，照片可以很好地提醒患者牙齿颜色的改变，避免不必要的纠纷。拍摄术前照片时可用比色板做参照，术后患者看到比色板色号的变化时，就会认识到自己牙齿的变化。

10. 漂白治疗应拍摄的照片

治疗前和治疗后应对比的内容如下。

（1）患者正面照。

（2）微笑照。

（3）牵拉观。

（4）将比色板放置在左上颌尖牙位置，拍摄微笑照。

（5）前牙黑背景牵拉观。

11. 治疗计划讨论和知情同意

在开始任何牙科治疗前，医师均应与患者讨论治疗计划。患者可从电脑或手机屏幕上浏览到自己口腔的全部情况，医师可向患者展示口内照片、电子口扫数据、影像学检查数据和石膏模型等等。医师需要向患者详细说明治疗计划、治疗顺序以及后续可能出现的进一步治疗。沟通是双向的，患者有机会提出进一步的问题，明确治疗方案所涉及到的内容，尤其是涉及到家庭漂白术的部分。医师应与患者讨论治疗的益处和风险，以及治疗方案的优点和缺点，同时说明漂白治疗或替代疗法的方案。

必须获得患者书面签字的知情同意书，知情同意书一式两份，一份交给患者，一份保留在患者病历内。知情同意书中应包括所有可能的副作用。

12. 颜色评估和比色

漂白治疗前有许多方法进行比色，较为常用的是传统比色板和电子比色仪。传统比色板使用较为广泛，但是比较主观；电子比色仪较为精准可控，但是需要额外投放设备。

传统比色板的影响因素包括：比色时的自然光、牙齿的色调、牙齿的明度和牙齿的色度。

针对牙齿颜色和比色的研究是一个更为宽泛的课题，本文不做深入探讨。值得一提的是，临床操作中必须做到用且仅用一套比色系统，达到精准、熟练和

可复制的要求。（图 5-1~ 图 5-17 ）

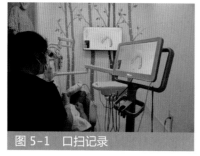

图 5-1　口扫记录

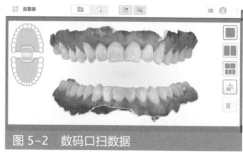

图 5-2　数码口扫数据

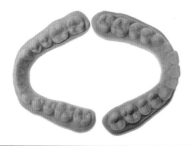

图 5-3　口扫数据三维打印模型 1

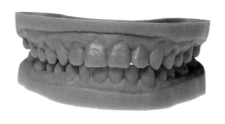

图 5-4　口扫数据三维打印模型 2

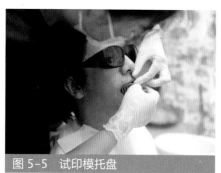

图 5-5　试印模托盘

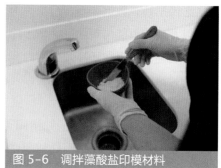

图 5-6　调拌藻酸盐印模材料

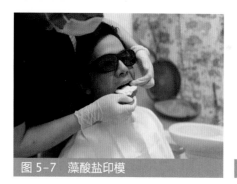

图 5-7　藻酸盐印模

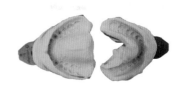

图 5-8　藻酸盐印模模型

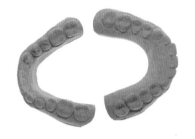

图 5-9　石膏研究模型 1

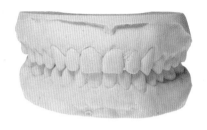

图 5-10　石膏研究模型 2

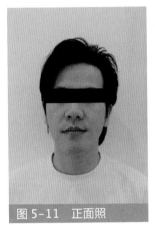

图 5-11　正面照

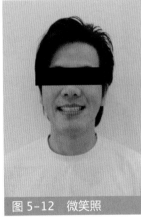

图 5-12　微笑照

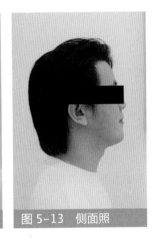

图 5-13　侧面照

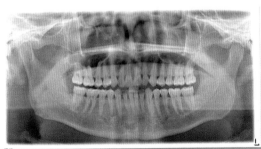

图 5-14　X 线曲面断层片

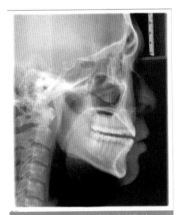

图 5-15　X 线头颅侧位片

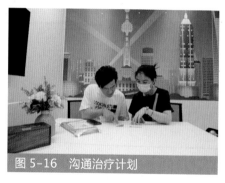

图 5-16　沟通治疗计划

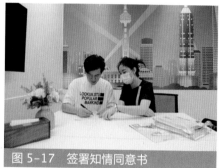

图 5-17　签署知情同意书

附：

XXXX 口腔门诊部

微笑评估表

1. 您是否喜欢目前牙齿的外观（大小和形态）？	是☐　否☐
2. 您是否满意目前牙齿的颜色？	是☐　否☐
3. 您是否希望牙齿变白？	是☐　否☐
4. 您对牙齿的整齐度是否满意？	是☐　否☐
5. 您是否有希望修复的缺失牙？	是☐　否☐
6. 您是否有希望更换的修复体（银汞充填体 / 金属冠）？	是☐　否☐

7. 如果可以任意改变自己的微笑，您希望具体做出那些改变？
具体：

新患者检查前问卷

初诊时间：_____年____月____日

姓名：_____

出生日期：_____年____月____日　　性别：□男　□女

联系方式：_____

主诉：	
您希望解决哪些牙齿问题：	
您希望接受哪些治疗：	
您对医师的希望和要求：	
与治疗相关的焦虑和反感之处：	
既往牙科治疗史：	上一次看牙：
	定期随访：
	具体治疗：
是否疼痛（具体性质）：	
是否敏感（具体诱因）：	□热　□冷　□甜　□压力　其他：_____
牙龈问题：	□出血　□结石　□红肿　□退缩　其他：_____
既往口腔卫生维护治疗：	
笑线和唇线：	
您最喜欢自己微笑的哪方面？	
您最不喜欢自己微笑的哪方面？	
您希望改善哪些方面？	
您是否对牙齿颜色感到满意？	

您是否希望牙齿内收或变直？	
您是否有希望关闭的牙齿间隙？	
您是否对牙齿的整齐度满意？	
您是否对牙齿的形态满意？	
您是否有希望修复的缺失牙？	
您是否有希望更换的修复体 （银汞充填体 / 金属冠）？	

牙齿：

既往正畸治疗史：	
食物嵌塞：	
智齿：	
颞下颌关节：	□弹响　□磨牙症　□牙关紧闭　□手术
其他补充事项：	

检查、诊断

患者详细信息：

姓名：	性别：□男　□女	出生日期：
移动电话：	邮箱：	微信：
对牙齿漂白的预期和要求：		
全身病史（用药史）：		

牙齿变色诊断：

变色类型：	轻度	中度	重度

目前颜色：	期望颜色：
□白垩斑	□氟斑牙
□褐斑	□四环素牙
□脱水线	□暗色裂纹

其他：

牙齿敏感：□是　□否	牙齿敏感治疗史：□是　□否

影像学检查和牙齿照片：

影像拍摄日期：	影像阅读日期：	

□根尖片	□全景片	□侧位片	□ CBCT
□口内照　拍摄日期：		□口外照　拍摄日期：	

牙髓活力测试：

口内检查：

牙龈退缩：

需要治疗：

旧修复体：

牙周疾病：□是　□否

患者需要进一步修复治疗，具体如下：

医师签名：	日期：

牙齿漂白处方

漂白治疗类型：	基础	中级	高级

全身病史回顾日期：		用药史回顾日期：	
目前口内情况：		术前告知检查情况：	

前牙充填体：		牙龈情况：	牙龈退缩：
全冠：		白垩斑：	暗色裂纹：
种植体全冠：		褐斑：	牙齿敏感：
贴面：		旧充填体：	脱水线：
其他：		修复体：	四环素牙：
		氟斑牙：	其他：
诊室漂白：		家庭漂白：	

牙齿漂白治疗产品：

产品名称	
产品浓度	
脱敏剂	
免责声明	
日期	

患者知情并同意治疗：

患者签字：	日期：

治疗记录：

就诊次数：	复诊时间：

治疗计划：

最后一次就诊日期：	最终照片拍摄日期：

最终颜色：

牙齿漂白术
患者知情同意书 / 健康诊疗记录表

日期：_____ / ___ /　　　　　　　　　病历号：_____

姓名：_____

出生日期：_____年___月___日　　　　性别：□男　□女

联系方式：_____

地址：_____

职业：_____

电子邮件：_____

紧急联系人：_____

请关注下列问题：

您的眼睛对各种光源敏感吗？　　　　　　　　　　　□是　□否

您的皮肤很容易被晒伤吗？　　　　　　　　　　　　□是　□否

您现在怀孕吗？　　　　　　　　　　　　　　　　　□是　□否

请仔细阅读以下内容：

1. 专业冷光牙齿漂白术适用人群

想改变牙齿颜色的人均可接受冷光牙齿漂白术治疗，但不建议 16 岁以下儿童及孕妇接受该治疗。根据牙齿变色的原因不同，医生将为您制定合理、完整的治疗计划。

2. 漂白效果

专业牙齿漂白术的效果十分显著，但是牙齿变色的原因有很多种，很难十分确定地预测您的牙齿能够漂白到何种程度，黄色或黄棕色牙齿的漂白效果一般来说会比灰色和灰棕色的漂白效果快且好。因服用抗生素、服用四环素、根管治疗或外伤性引起的牙齿变色以及牙面上的白色斑点，可能需要一次以上的漂白疗程。在咨询过程中，医生会向您展示从前病例漂白前、后的照片，以增加您对本公司牙齿漂白产品治疗效果的认知，医生也会根据您的牙齿状况来评估您的牙齿可能达到的漂白效果。如果您有任何疑问，请在签名或接受漂白治疗前，和您的医生讨论确认，每位患者都应按医生提出的治疗建议完成牙齿漂白过程。

3. 保养维护

在牙齿漂白后的 24~48 小时之间，牙齿的漂白效果会变得更加均匀，牙齿也更富有光泽，这是因为牙齿表面会重新形成保护膜。此外，您每天的饮食习惯也会形成牙齿的再染色，再染色的状况会因吸烟和食用咖啡、茶、槟榔、红酒等有色饮食的多少而定。可以自行在家以自助式的"家庭牙齿漂白术"进行居家漂白和保养，使漂白效果更加持久和稳定。

4. 潜在的问题与风险

任何形式的美学治疗在操作过程中都存在着程度不一的风险和限制。虽然专业的牙齿漂白术极少发生问题与危险（即使存在、程度也非常轻），但是我们希望您能事先了解可能潜在的问题与风险。请详细阅读以下信息，如果有任何疑问，请在签名之前和您的医生确认。

（1）牙齿敏感：在牙齿漂白疗程中，部分人士由于牙齿存在隐裂、磨耗、缺损等问题可能感觉到轻微的牙齿酸痛，如果您的牙齿平时出现过敏感现象，请在治疗前告知，我们会调整漂白剂量和光源照射时间，以减轻您的不适，但是我们无法完全避免敏感酸疼现象。针对某些牙齿敏感的特例，我们建议患者在疗程前服用环氧化酶抑制剂。若您在疗程中感到任何不舒服，请及时通知医生，我们会做一些调整以减轻您的不适。牙齿漂白后的轻微酸痛感通常在 12~24 小时自行消除。

（2）牙龈和口腔组织不适：在疗程中可能出现暂时性的灼热，一般是因为口腔组织接触到漂白剂，我们会为您涂抹牙龈保护剂，尽可能避免这些情况发生，保护您的口腔组织。此外，为了达到最好的漂白效果，我们将使用开口器撑开您的嘴唇，因此您可能感到轻微的不适，这类的不适在漂白治疗结束后会消除。大部分病人在治疗过程中不会产生不适感，如果您的口腔有不舒服的感觉，请以温水漱口。

（3）树脂充填、义齿、瓷贴面、修复体、金属冠等无法通过这种漂白治疗改变颜色，漂白的结果和天然牙颜色不同，我们将尽可能为您消除义齿上的色素和斑点。所有修复过的牙齿、义齿和树脂填充物等，可能会与漂白后的天然牙颜色不同，请在疗程进行前，和您的医生进行沟通。

5. 您的权益

为了确保漂白效果及维护您的健康，漂白前请务必确认您的一次性牙齿漂白剂包装未经开封。

授权书：

本人在这份文件中提供的资料正确无误。

本人已经详细阅读完并理解以上的信息，对于牙科及其所提供的服务，本人已经有完全的了解，所有本人的疑问已经获得该机构专业人员的完整回答，本人对所获得的信息和回答感到满意。

基于以上的认知，本人授权牙科以及该机构专业医疗人员为本人实施牙齿漂白治疗术及相关疗程，并同意支付所有费用。

客户签名：＿＿＿＿＿＿＿＿　　　　医生签名：＿＿＿＿＿＿＿＿＿

日期：＿＿＿＿＿＿＿＿＿　　　　　日期：＿＿＿＿＿＿＿＿＿＿

第六章
诊室漂白治疗步骤

 防范说明和副作用的处理

1. 无局部麻醉，患者监控

牙齿漂白术不应进行局部麻醉。医师应全程监控，以便及时发现牙齿不适症状。应指导患者在出现任何烧灼、刺痛或不适感时及时举手示意或按警示铃。若患者出现牙齿敏感且无法缓解，应立刻终止治疗！

2. 牙齿敏感

在初诊和术前检查时筛选出合适的患者，将使牙齿敏感发生的可能性降至最低。牙齿敏感的一些危险因素包括龋坏、牙龈退缩、颈部缺损和牙齿敏感病史。对于牙齿敏感病史的患者，有3个解决方案：①术前2周连续使用含硝酸钾牙膏或脱敏剂，缓解不适；②高风险患者术前30分钟服用环氧化酶抑制剂或相关止痛片；③漂白术中，舌侧应用3%~6%硝酸钾凝胶同步抗敏。

3. 软组织灼伤或唇肿胀

一定要小心仔细地涂布牙龈保护剂，若漂白剂从牙龈保护剂下方发生渗漏，或意外接触到软组织，则需要立刻用大量清水冲洗，并涂布油脂，如维生素E、凡士林等。油脂可缓解软组织刺痛症状，软组织苍白现象会在数小时内缓解。可给予患者一些凡士林或表面麻醉剂，供患者回家后使用。若患者皮肤发生过敏反应，应考虑使用抗组胺药物。

4. 白垩斑

治疗前应尽可能发现所有的白垩斑，因为在漂白治疗中，脱水会让白垩斑更加明显。治疗后 24 小时内，这些白垩斑会随着牙齿再水化逐渐淡化。

5. 光敏感

医师在使用漂白冷光仪前，应明确患者是否在服用含有光敏感的药物，或患者是否患有光敏感性皮肤疾病，是否可能出现皮肤不良反应，如唇和周围组织的肿胀。

6. 孕期或哺乳期女性及未成年儿童

我们建议推迟孕期或哺乳期女性及未成年儿童的治疗。

二　洁治

漂白前的准备工作，应使用橡皮杯或纤维刷蘸取抛光膏或浮石粉清洁牙面色素、菌斑等。（图 6-1~ 图 6-7）

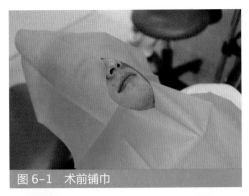

图 6-1　术前铺巾

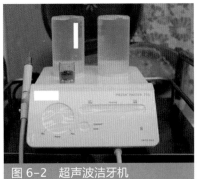

图 6-2　超声波洁牙机

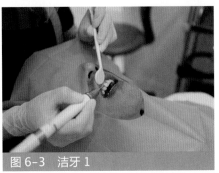

图 6-3　洁牙 1

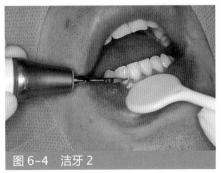

图 6-4　洁牙 2

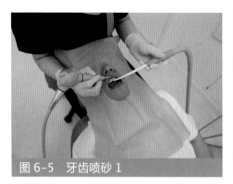

图 6-5　牙齿喷砂 1

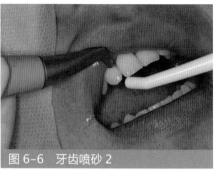

图 6-6　牙齿喷砂 2

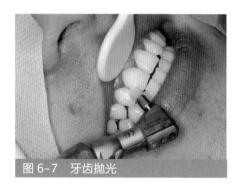

图 6-7　牙齿抛光

三　术前比色和照相

在自然光下，用视觉比色法或电子比色仪记录术前牙齿颜色。术后患者通常会忘记术前牙齿颜色，术前比色板的记录有助于展示治疗后牙齿颜色的改善。（图 6-8~ 图 6-11）

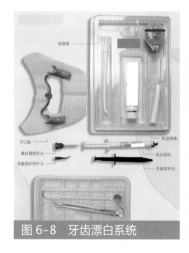

图 6-8　牙齿漂白系统

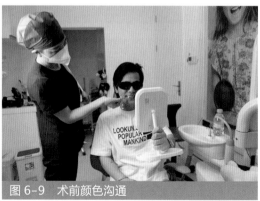

图 6-9　术前颜色沟通

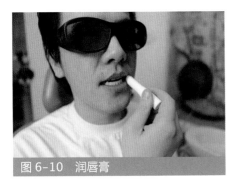

图 6-10　润唇膏

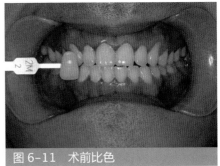

图 6-11　术前比色

四　护目镜和光罩

　　使用漂白冷光仪器时，必须为患者佩戴护目镜或洞巾，避免对眼球造成损伤。同时建议在光照出口处加装柔光罩，避免有害光线散射。

五　唇颊牵拉和保护

　　医师应给患者唇部涂布唇膏保护嘴唇，维生素 E 和凡士林是一种脂溶性抗氧化剂，可中和过氧化物对软组织的意外损伤。有多种唇颊侧开口器适合治疗使用，建议使用带舌档的开口器；同时将铺巾放在开口器下方，进一步保护口周软组织。（图 6-12~图 6-13）

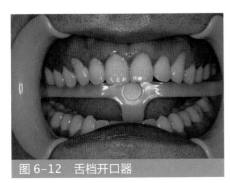

图 6-12　舌档开口器

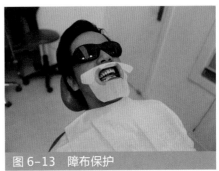

图 6-13　障布保护

六　保护牙周软组织

　　开口器就位后，在前庭沟内放置隔湿棉卷；吹干龈沟液，用输送管沿牙龈边缘小心涂布光固化牙龈保护剂，避免牙龈发生化学灼伤；也可以将牙龈保护剂向根方延伸 5~10mm，与隔湿棉卷接触，形成一个整体，封闭牙龈。使用光固化灯，每个牙位光照约 10 秒，使牙龈保护剂完全固化。注意，光固化灯应该保持移动，因为功率过高的光固化灯可引起软组织不适。（图 6-14~ 图 6-19）

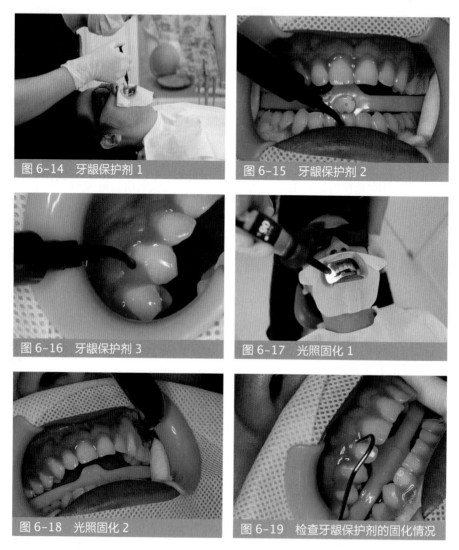

图 6-14　牙龈保护剂 1

图 6-15　牙龈保护剂 2

图 6-16　牙龈保护剂 3

图 6-17　光照固化 1

图 6-18　光照固化 2

图 6-19　检查牙龈保护剂的固化情况

七　激活漂白剂

　　双注射器混合型漂白剂需将含漂白剂的注射器与含激活剂的注射剂混合，并排尽气泡。冰箱内储存的漂白剂需要提前放置室温，或在热水浴内预热。

八　涂布漂白剂

　　将漂白剂涂布到牙齿上，厚度 1~2mm，通常反应 15~20 分钟，每次就诊重复 2 次。重复涂布漂白剂前，应用外科吸引装置吸尽旧漂白剂。若患者出现任何疼痛症状，应立即吸走所有漂白剂，并用大量水冲洗。若隔湿棉卷过湿，则应该及时更换。（图 6-20~ 图 6-25）

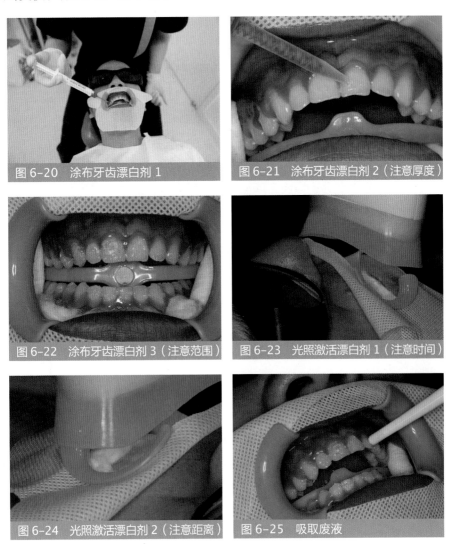

图 6-20　涂布牙齿漂白剂 1

图 6-21　涂布牙齿漂白剂 2（注意厚度）

图 6-22　涂布牙齿漂白剂 3（注意范围）

图 6-23　光照激活漂白剂 1（注意时间）

图 6-24　光照激活漂白剂 2（注意距离）

图 6-25　吸取废液

九　去除牙龈保护剂

在漂白治疗结束后，应用探针整块去除牙龈保护剂，注意不要遗漏。

十　术后比色

采用相同的比色系统进行术后比色，并且记录在案，向患者展示术后的即刻效果。（图 6-26~图 6-30）

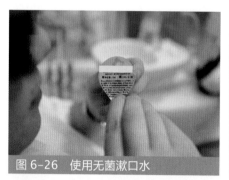

图 6-26　使用无菌漱口水

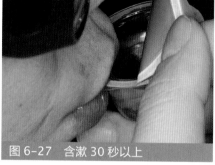

图 6-27　含漱 30 秒以上

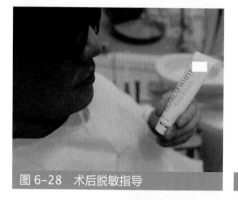

图 6-28　术后脱敏指导

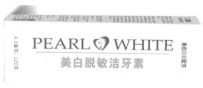

图 6-29　美白脱敏洁牙素

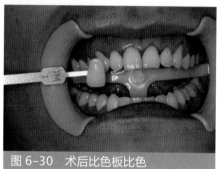

图 6-30　术后比色板比色

术后指导

术后指导意见包括但不局限于：至少 1 周内不要饮用含色素的饮品，例如咖啡、茶叶和葡萄酒等；术前需要使用脱敏剂或止痛片的患者，术后继续使用有助于缓解牙齿敏感；为了保持漂白效果，可使用家庭漂白术联合治疗，定期维护。（图 6-31~ 图 6-32 ）

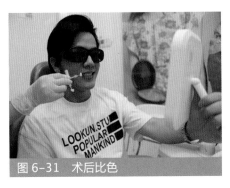

图 6-31　术后比色

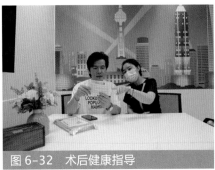

图 6-32　术后健康指导

第七章
家庭漂白治疗步骤

家庭漂白术是一项较为简化的治疗技术，患者与医师初步沟通后，获得个性化定制的牙套或漂白托盘进行居家漂白。医师将家庭漂白剂交给患者，并附加详细的使用方案。本章节详细描述家庭漂白技术及方法，帮助医师获得成功的疗效。

一　防范说明和副作用的处理

医师应当详细明确该技术的优缺点，便于和患者沟通。

1. 优点

（1）简单快速，易于实施。

（2）椅旁时间短。

（3）性价比高。

（4）牙齿敏感性低。

（5）患者治疗时间自由度高。

2. 缺点

（1）依赖于患者的配合度。

（2）牙齿漂白的疗效取决于反应时间。若患者戴用牙套和漂白剂时间不满足要求，疗效会降低。

（3）存在滥用的可能性。

（4）口腔异物敏感性高的患者难以配合。

其余步骤包括但不局限于：初诊问诊，口腔常规检查，术前比色评估，照相和制定完整计划等，与"诊室漂白术"相仿。

二　印模

应制取精细印模，复制出上下颌牙齿形态，或口扫记录上下颌牙齿数据，便于制作漂白托盘和个性化牙套。取模使用藻酸盐，调拌材料时，应尽可能排净气泡；口扫时，应用气枪吹干唾液，以获得良好细节。

三　模型

模型的制作特别重要，口扫数据可以委托义齿加工中心 3D 打印后，直接制作个性化牙套；藻酸盐印模材料应当尽快灌制模型，避免变形。应将上下颌模型修整为马鞍形，保留上颌和下颌的牙齿及牙周组织，不包括颚部及舌侧组织。模型应基底平坦，与中切牙保持垂直，这样使得真空压制的牙套更易于模型贴合，避免加工过程中形成各种皱褶。

四　制作个性化牙套

通常委托义齿加工中心制作个性化牙套，也可在门诊部的加工室自行制作。有些医师习惯在牙齿模型的唇颊侧预留空间，制作储药池，但并无研究表明这样可以加速漂白过程；推测无论有无储药池，漂白剂降解的速率都是一样的。但储药池也有一些优点，如增加牙套的固位、减少对牙龈的过度挤压等。

五　试戴牙套和患者指导

先指导患者在口内试戴牙套，若发现牙套边缘覆盖牙龈超过 1mm 以上，需打磨光滑，避免牙套边缘对口腔软组织造成刺激。教会患者如何摘戴牙套、如何放置漂白剂。

六　医嘱

漂白剂用量应适当，勿溢出牙齿范围，触及牙龈，如有溢出应及时去除，以防吞咽；每次的戴用时间应按照产品操作指南执行；每次漂白完成后应及时冲洗、擦干牙套，存放在牙套盒内保存；出现牙齿过敏、牙龈炎症时，停戴 1~2 天，并与医师联系；牙齿漂白期间建议使用含氟牙膏刷牙。

七 疗程

总的疗程需要根据实际情况灵活制定，一般需要 1~6 个月。请患者每 2 周复诊 1 次，了解患者的操作是否正确，检查牙色改变状况、牙龈有无炎症、牙套有无缺损等，发现问题后应及时解决。

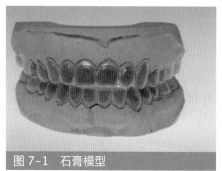

图 7-1　石膏模型

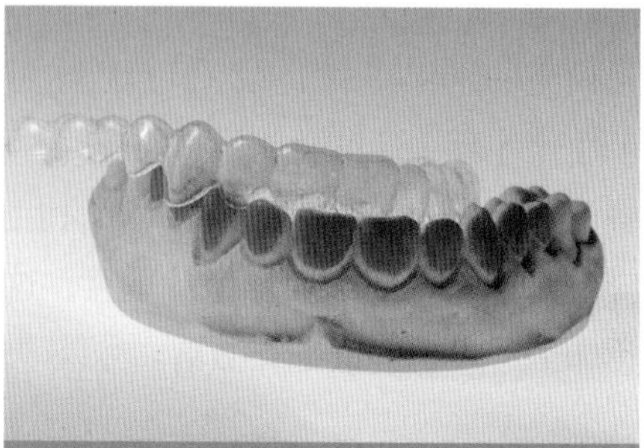

图 7-2　红色树脂：储药囊

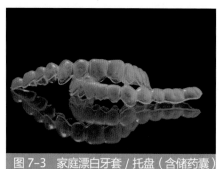

图 7-3　家庭漂白牙套/托盘（含储药囊）

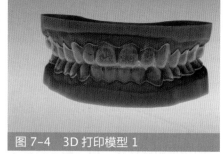

图 7-4　3D 打印模型 1

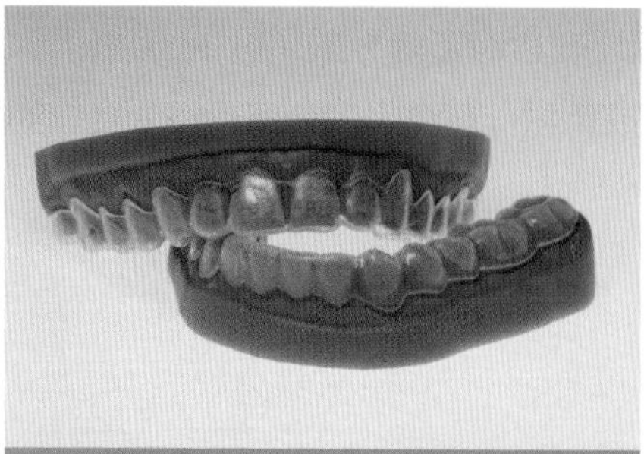

图 7-5　3D 打印模型 2

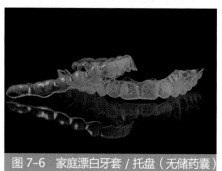

图 7-6　家庭漂白牙套/托盘（无储药囊）

一 牙根外吸收

　　牙根外吸收是无髓牙内漂白技术的主要并发症，发生率为7%，原因不完全清楚。过去的临床研究表明，出现牙根外吸收的患者年龄大多集中在25岁以下，且牙齿变色原因多为牙外伤。动物实验显示，使用热催化法发生牙根外吸收的概率为18%~25%，而不用热催化法者的概率为0%~6%。推测牙根外吸收的发生机制可能是强氧化剂经过无牙骨质覆盖的牙本质小管（约10%的牙齿存在这种解剖缺陷）或有缺陷的牙骨质渗透到牙周，引起牙骨质坏死及牙周膜炎症，感染使炎症症状持续，最终导致牙根外吸收。使用封闭性强的材料垫底以形成保护层、用过硼酸钠等弱氧化剂代替强氧化剂及不使用热催化技术等，也许会减少此类并发症的发生。

二 牙齿敏感

　　牙齿敏感是活髓牙外漂白技术的主要并发症，约60%的患者会出现轻微而短暂的牙齿敏感症状，但一般不会对牙髓造成实质性损伤，终止治疗后基本可恢复。为减少牙齿敏感症状的发生，可于漂白术前和术后使用氟化物。

三 软组织损伤

　　诊室内使用的高浓度过氧化氢容易造成软组织烧伤，烧伤深度通常较浅，使用大量水冲洗后在创面涂布防腐抗炎类药物，通常会很快恢复，不会产生后遗症。家庭漂白时出现的软组织损伤多为不合适的牙套或托盘所致，正常剂量的漂白剂不会造成明显的软组织损伤。

四 釉质表面的影响

研究表明，漂白剂会造成釉质表面显微硬度下降，但漂白使用氟化物可以促进再矿化。漂白过程会释放很多氧到牙齿中，抑制了树脂的聚合，因此漂白后等待 1~2 周时间可以让这种副作用减弱，不仅能获得良好的粘接效果，还可以保证比色时牙齿颜色更稳定。

五 漂白药物对常见充填材料的影响

1. 对复合树脂的影响

漂白剂会增加树脂表面的粗糙度和硬度，但并无临床意义；漂白剂接触树脂材料后，对其颜色并无显著改变，但会使树脂边缘的微渗漏增加。

2. 对其他修复材料的影响

漂白剂对瓷和金没有影响，对某些银汞合金会促进汞的释放，但无临床意义；此外，漂白剂会使甲基丙烯酸甲酯的临时冠变色，通过改变玻璃离子水门汀中的基质结构而影响其功能。

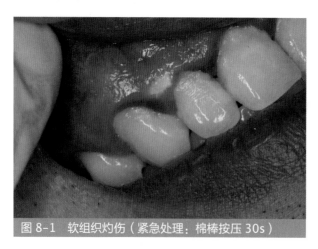

图 8-1 软组织灼伤（紧急处理：棉棒按压 30s）

第九章
特殊病例

 四环素牙

四环素类广谱抗生素于 1948 年问世，很快被应用于多种儿童及成人感染性疾病的治疗。所有四环素类化合物均包含 4 个相融的环状结构，因此得名四环素。使用四环素最明显的副作用是导致用药时发生矿化的组织内出现荧光色素沉积。四环素能够螯合钙离子，被牙齿、软骨和骨吸收，形成四环素 – 钙磷复合物，若在牙齿发育期间用药，可导致乳恒牙列牙齿变色、釉质发育不全。

1. 四环素牙的美学治疗的若干方案

（1）仅牙齿漂白。

（2）牙齿漂白结合复合树脂充填，覆盖变色区域。

（3）联合治疗：牙齿漂白 + 直接贴面法（无创贴面）。

（4）间接贴面法修复（有创贴面）。

（5）全冠修复。

不同的方法适用于不同程度的四环素牙，原则上应该以侵入性、创伤性最小的治疗手段作为首选，本章节主要讨论牙齿漂白术的问题。

2. 对四环素牙变色程度的分类及建议

（1）Ⅰ度：轻度四环素牙。黄色至灰色均匀变色，无条带样改变。

（2）Ⅱ度：中度四环素牙。黄褐色至深灰色变色。

（3）Ⅲ度：重度四环素牙。蓝灰色或黑色变色，伴明显条带。

（4）Ⅳ度：难处理病例，漂白通常无效。

（5）Ⅴ度：严重变色，釉质缺损，非适应证。

一般情况下，Ⅰ～Ⅲ度四环素牙漂白治疗有效，最佳选择是先进行漂白治疗，随后评估是否需要进一步进行侵入性更大的治疗。

3. 四环素牙漂白治疗方法

（1）长期家庭漂白，远期效果佳。

（2）家庭漂白和诊室漂白联合治疗。

（3）意向性根管治疗后内漂白。这种方法过于激进，争议很大，目前基本不建议使用。

二 氟牙症

氟牙症是地区慢性氟中毒的一个突出的症状。地区性慢性氟中毒是一种地方病，主要累及骨骼和发育期的牙齿。出现骨病变的严重慢性氟中毒，被称为氟骨症；而仅出现牙齿病变的慢性氟中毒，则被称为氟牙症。氟牙症是一种特殊类型的釉质发育不全，患牙在临床上主要表现为釉质上出现着色的斑块和缺损，所以又称为氟斑牙或斑釉牙。

氟牙症是一种地方病，氟牙症集中分布的地区称为氟牙症流行区。在氟牙症的临床和流行病学调查中常用的氟牙症分类为 Dean 分类法，于 1942 年提出，最早用于氟牙症的分类调查，也是世界卫生组织推荐使用的氟牙症分类标准：

（1）正常：釉质表面光滑，有光泽，通常呈乳白色。

（2）可疑：釉质的半透明度有轻度改变，从少数白斑纹到偶见白色斑点。

（3）很轻：小的呈纸样白色不透明区，不规则地分布在牙面上，但不超过牙面的 25%。

（4）轻度：牙面上的白色不透明区更广泛，但不超过牙面的 50%。

（5）中度：釉质表面有显著的磨损，呈黄褐色或棕褐色。

（6）重度：釉质表面严重受累，明显发育不全，棕褐染色广泛，影响到整个牙的外形。

一般情况下，轻度而无明显缺损的患牙可漂白治疗，或联合微研磨技术和渗透树脂技术。中度和重度有缺损的患牙建议使用陶瓷修复手段。

三　无髓牙

无髓牙漂白技术主要应用于改善外伤或牙髓治疗后引起变色的牙齿，虽然目前临床上应对无髓牙通常采用全瓷/锆冠修复治疗，但是仍然有一部分病例需要漂白治疗。该手段临床疗效不持久，颜色恢复率为83%~91%，治疗后1~5年，50%~65%的患牙可出现程度不同的颜色回退。我们本章节主要介绍冠内漂白法。

冠内漂白法是无髓牙漂白技术的常用方法，使用高浓度的漂白剂，必须在诊室操作。方法分为两种，即热催化法和渐进漂白法。热催化法是在30分钟内将放入髓腔内的22%~35%的过氧化氢加热数次，然后进行彻底冲洗，优点是疗效高、疗程短，缺点是易引起牙根外吸收，目前临床使用较少。渐进漂白法每次就诊时间短，且较安全，但疗程相对较长，是临床常用技术，操作步骤如下。

（1）完善根管治疗：漂白治疗前，必须拍摄 X 线片，确认根管已做过完善的根管充填。

（2）安装橡皮障，保护牙龈不被强氧化剂烧伤。

（3）髓腔清理：使用慢速球钻清除髓腔内容物，揭净髓顶，确保髓角及其他可能隐藏牙髓组织的区域充分暴露。髓腔内有树脂充填体时更应仔细清理，切勿残留树脂材料，以便使漂白剂能与牙本质紧密接触并有效渗透。

（4）垫底：去除部分根充物，用磷酸锌水门汀或玻璃离子水门汀等材料垫底，以形成保护层，阻止漂白剂向根方渗透。垫底材料的厚度至少2mm，冠方高度与牙龈的附着上皮一致，以使漂白剂能渗入牙颈部"S"形的牙本质小管，脱去牙冠部的颜色。

（5）置入漂白剂：将高浓度过氧化氢溶液直接放入髓腔。为安全起见，也可使用过硼酸钠与水/生理盐水调和成糊状或10%过氧化脲放入髓腔。

（6）髓腔封闭：用黏性较强的封闭剂封堵漂白剂，如玻璃离子或树脂等，避免漂白剂泄露。

（7）复诊：根据所用漂白剂的不同，确定复诊的间隔时间。每次复诊时均应记录牙齿颜色，复诊次数依颜色的变化而定，一般需3~6次。漂白完成时的牙色应略白于同颌同名牙，给牙色回退留以空间；若牙色经多次复诊后未达到预定目标，且颜色已无明显变化时，应征求患者意见，终止漂白治疗，按照需求做修复治疗。

（8）完成：漂白治疗终止后2周，用合适牙色的复合树脂充填髓腔。

第十章
术后管理

在前面的章节我们都强调了术前沟通和规范治疗计划的重要性，术后管理主要也是围绕这个中心思想展开的，主要涉及到 3 个方面：治疗的持久性、治疗后的副作用和安全问题。

一 持久性

该话题是患者最关注的问题，尽管很多文献和宣传都强调了漂白治疗术后"持续性"和"满意度"很高，但是由于各个专家学者的评判标准不尽相同，故不可"神话"牙齿漂白术的持久性。

第一个问题"漂白效果能够维持多久"。客观认知先从文献入手，1990 年 Van Haywood 医师对患者队列随访 12 年：74% 在术后 1.5 年对颜色满意，术后 3 年满意率降低至 62%。2002 年 Ritter 医师对患者队列随访 9~12 年结果：平均治疗 10 年后颜色保持率和满意率为 43%。2011 年 Leonard 随访 47 个月报告表示，89% 的患者仍然保持美白效果，82% 患者牙齿颜色仍较基准线至少改善 2 个色号，平均颜色改善 5 个 Vita 比色板单位。

第二个问题"是否需要再次漂白，如果需要，频率是什么"。1994 年 Haywood 研究报告，在治疗后平均 25 个月需进行再次漂白；2011 年 Leonard 研究报告再次漂白发生在第 32 个月。

还有一个核心因素就是患者的术后饮食结构，不同的操作指南对于术后即刻的饮食会有不同的要求，主要集中于术后至少 6 小时 ~2 周不要饮用任何有颜色的饮料，这一点争议较大。

综上所述，我们给出的建议是：①漂白治疗后颜色维持的时间为 1.5~2 年；②再次漂白即润色漂白的最高频率为 7 天后；③至少在漂白术后的 48~72 小时内不要饮用任何有颜色的饮料。

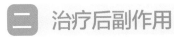

二　治疗后副作用

如之前的章节所述，漂白术后主要副作用为牙龈刺激和牙齿敏感 2 个问题。

1. 牙龈刺激主要发生在家庭漂白术中

最可能的原因是托盘边缘伸展至牙龈，漂白剂在牙龈边缘潴留。可以通过修剪牙套边缘来解决这个问题，即使牙套没有完全覆盖整个牙面，随着时间的推移和漂白剂在釉柱间的渗透，牙齿也可以整体变白。

2. 牙齿敏感有多种原因

首先应排除术中操作不规范或过度脱水导致的问题；其次考虑牙套的软硬程度和贴合程度，是否产生了"正畸力量"；第三评估家庭漂白剂浓度的选择，是否增加了敏感风险。建议术前居家连续使用 2 周含硝酸钾和氟化物的牙膏制品；在术前使用 3% 硝酸钾和 0.11% 氟化物脱敏剂 30 分钟以上；家庭漂白期间坚持使用脱敏制剂。

同时应该向患者强调术后饮食结构的重要性，控制柠檬类酸性水果及果汁、可乐等碳酸饮料和槟榔类坚硬食物的食用。

三　安全问题

牙齿漂白术后的患者并未经常出现副作用，如龋坏、牙齿折断、口腔病理变化或牙髓病理变化等。一般来说，漂白术后唯一的长期改变是牙齿颜色术后即刻变浅。牙齿漂白术的有效性和安全性均与其他规范牙科治疗手段相同。

主要参考文献

［1］樊明文，周学东. 牙体牙髓病学［M］. 北京：人民卫生出版社，2016.

［2］高学军，岳林. 牙体牙髓病学［M］. 北京：北京大学出版社，2017.

［3］Linda Greenwall，刘擎，周锐（译）. 牙齿美白 Tooth Whitening Techniques ［M］. 沈阳：辽宁科技出版社，2020.

特别致谢

致谢牙齿漂白系统的挚友，给我提供了宝贵的在漂白剂实验室和产品加工中心的学习机会。

特别鸣谢：沈健

致谢门诊部工作同事提供的拍摄场地和帮助。

特别鸣谢：龙芸、杨芳霞、邱萍

致谢义齿加工中心提供了 3D 打印和个性化漂白牙套的制作和帮助。

特别鸣谢：王恒、龚证

致谢在齿科医师工作中对我有帮助和启发的医师。

特别鸣谢：沈华、孔晔

致谢愿意分享自己牙齿漂白经验的患者，患者是医师最好的老师！